D1025024

BLACK BIRD FLY AWAY

DISABLED IN AN ABLE-BODIED WORLD

BLACK BIRD FLY AWAY

DISABLED IN AN ABLE-BODIED WORLD

HUGH GREGORY GALLAGHER

FOREWORD BY GEOFFREY C. WARD

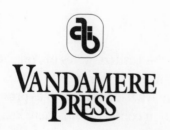

VANDAMERE
PRESS

Published by
Vandamere Press
P.O. Box 5243
Arlington, VA 22205

Copyright 1998
Vandamere Press

ISBN 0-918339-44-8

"As I see it, it is through the process of making—
plays, poems, novels—out of one's experience that
one becomes a writer, and it is through this
process, this struggle, that the writer helps give
meaning to the experience of his group."

Ralph Ellison
Author, *Invisible Man*

CONTENTS

FOREWORD

BY GEOFFREY C. WARD

THIS IS A TOUGH, honest invaluable book by a tough, honest, invaluable man. I've known Hugh Gallagher for thirteen years now. We have at least three things in common. We both were hit by infantile paralysis in the early 1950's (he with much more devastating impact than I, as his harrowing account included here makes clear). We have both written extensively about Franklin Roosevelt and the impact polio had on him. And we are both currently learning to cope with the effects of post-polio syndrome, the near-extinct disease's last bitter joke on those of us who dared to think they'd conquered it. Not long ago I consulted Hugh about the maddeningly conflicting advice given to those of us on whom the joke has been played: some doctors warn against exercise for fear of further exhausting already-depleted muscles; others suggest keeping surviving muscles strong with hearty workouts. "Listen to your body," Hugh told me the last time I muttered to him about it all. "And remember, whatever you choose to do will turn out to have been wrong."

Gallows humor like that is typical of polios and Hugh is a master of it. But nothing could have prepared me for the power of this collection of pieces written over the past 40 years.

Gallagher's unflinching memories of first contracting polio, then almost losing the struggle against its initial onslaught, and finally being forced to make the emotional and physical adjustments dictated by paraplegia, are unforgettable. They are also hard reading for anyone who, like me, struggled to bury all the feelings the author dredges up with such pitiless candor: the pain and anger, the humiliation and frustration and depression; above all, the desperate need to mask one's own terror of helplessness by constantly assuring the rest of the world that everything's just dandy.

It is impossible for anyone not to admire Hugh Gallagher's gallantry—a word I'm sure he'll hate having applied to him—or his extraordinary achievements in and out of the corridors of power in Washington, or his hard-won triumph over the depression that threatened to cripple him as even polio never could.

Disabled people will draw sustenance from this book but I also can't imagine a more useful volume for any able bodied person— parent or child, spouse or companion, friend or relation—who wants to understand what the disabled really feel about the challenges brought by each new day.

BLACK BIRD FLY AWAY

DISABLED IN AN ABLE-BODIED WORLD

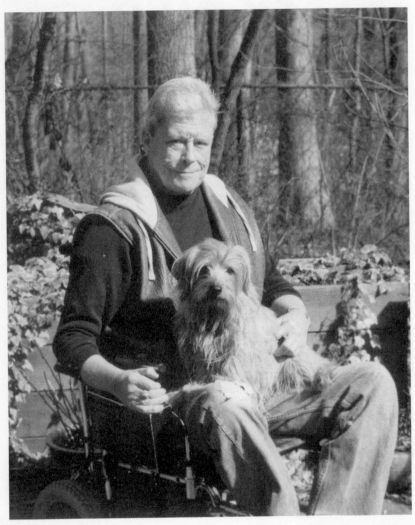

photo by John Holstein

This Thing Has a Happy Ending ... Right?

MEDICAL HISTORY TELLS of an American Indian who had a bullet wound in his stomach that never healed. By looking through the hole in the Indian's stomach, doctors for the first time were able to see how the stomach digests food. Curiously, this wound is what it is like to be disabled. I'm not sure our wounds ever heal either.

I am a polio quadriplegic who has used a wheelchair for some forty years. Over this period, the physical and social aspects of being disabled have greatly improved. In the social terms of the 1950s, to be paralyzed and "confined" to a wheelchair was thought to be—as it was—an appalling catastrophe. Until the development and widespread use of antibiotics and other treatments in the years following World War II, the life expectancy of a quadriplegic was not long. Pneumonia, kidney and bladder infections, pressure sores, and other such afflictions made life short and painful.

Forty years ago, most people were uncomfortable in the presence of the disabled. When I went out in public in my wheelchair, I could sense their embarrassment. And their discomfort would of course, make me uncomfortable. The environment was filled with obstacles for someone like me in a wheelchair—entrances were inaccessible, stairs were everywhere, and there were no curb cuts or convenient parking places. There were no public bathrooms I could use; I was kept off airplanes and out of theaters because of my chair. Education and employment were denied to many of my peers.

Today, things have changed on two fronts. First, it is a lot easier to be disabled. Disabled people are healthier and live longer, thanks to modern medicine. They are far more active. Because of efficient and dependable wheelchairs, long-life batteries, vans, wheelchair lifts, and a conscientious effort to make society physically accessible, disabled people are able to play a more visible and active role in the community. Second, this new visibility and activity, this new *viability,* has served to change social attitudes. Disability is no longer seen as the catastrophe it once was. There is a new awareness of our needs. Efforts to integrate the disabled into mainstream society have met with public support.

Timothy Nugent, who pioneered a program to enroll persons with severe disabilities as students at the University of Illinois after World War II, used to argue that the physical barrier *is* the disability. Remove the barrier—put in a ramp, widen a door, get a lift—and the disability no longer exists. Disability was a social, environmental problem, rather than a psychological and emotional trauma. I know disabled people who try very hard to believe this. Their belief allows them to externalize the anger they feel about their condition. They want to believe that it is the injustice of society that is the cause of the rage and frustration they feel.

My 40 years of experience tells me they are wrong. Disability is far more complex, more profound than mere physical impairment. The loss of mobility, function, sensation, or faculty involved with disability is only the physical aspect. In my experience the emotional aspects of the loss have a greater and more persistent impact. In those terms, nothing has changed in 40 years. It is the same old thing—a psychic wound that never heals. Like the stomach wound of the unfortunate

Indian, our wounds provide a window into the human condition. We see through our disability, just how very fragile and temporary is our hold on life, how insecure our physical strength and health.

Young Americans believe they are immortal; they are taught to believe they can grow up to be anything they want. Early on, people with disabilities find this is not so; they know that such talk is just whistling in the dark.

Through our disability, we are granted—if we can stand it—the despair *and* the wisdom that springs therefrom, usually reserved for the old and dying. We must live with this knowledge. Can a life—with its share of joy and reward—be wrested from this encompassing, ever-present knowledge?

In T.S. Eliot's *The Waste Land* there is the image of a ghostly presence, ". . . who walks always beside you/. . . There is always another one walking beside you . . ." In his notes, Eliot refers to the experience of Arctic explorer, Ernest Shackleton, who, close to death from cold and exhaustion, sensed a presence beside him. When he looked, there was no one but when he turned away, he again sensed the presence just beyond the periphery of his vision.

Just so for us. Amputees continue to sense the presence of the missing limb. The limb is gone but its ghost remains. And it is the same for paralyzed people. Within the crippled limb there remains the memory of the unimpaired one. Within the floppy Raggedy Ann body, there remains, like a memory, the able-bodied ghost of its former self.

How many times a day—in my mind's eye—I stand to reach a book on a high shelf, run to get the mail, jump into the shower. It happens every day, and every day I am forcibly reminded of my disability. After 40 years of paralysis the memory of movement is as strong today as it was before. The instinct to act even though action is impossible—it hangs on.

My old boss, Senator Bartlett, once recalled asking his mother what it was like to be 80. "It's the strangest thing," she replied, "I am the same young person I ever was but here I am, trapped inside this old, worn-out body." Disabled people understand.

Strange as it may be, I am both disabled and able-bodied at the same time. It might be expected that—over time—the inner ghost of the able-bodied me would fade as—over time—I learn to live with my disability. On the routine level of daily living, this is the case. But at a deeper and more important level, this is *not* the case. Over the years, my self image remains that of a nondisabled person, the ghost inside, while the frail and paralyzed person—my *real* and daily person—I seem to treat as an aberration, an inconvenience in my progress through life. Thus I admit my infirmity, drag it around with me, but it is not me. *I* am my ghost, a living dichotomy. I am an able-bodied idea inside a disabled reality. Can one live like this?

Franklin D. Roosevelt did it by denying the reality. In my book, *FDR's Splendid Deception*, I show the tremendous efforts made by President Roosevelt to appear able-bodied when he was, in fact, a paraplegic. These efforts were made not just to convince others but himself as well. Of all his many strengths, the most impressive by far was the sheer force of his determination, his absolute determination that he was in every significant way whole and fit. One senses that this conviction was as important to him as life itself.

This sort of thing can be effective, but it is exhausting and isolating. Take the crazy example of silent screen star Mary Pickford. She was determined to remain "America's Sweetheart," young and beautiful forever. As age overtook her, she retreated into seclusion, allowing no one to see her aged face. At dinner parties, she would converse with her guests by intercom from another room rather than expose her wrinkles to view.

Flat denial of hard reality can serve a useful purpose—it buys time for coming to terms with trauma. Modern medical rehabilitation theory holds that, while temporary denial is normal, continued denial is unhealthy. Over time, according to theory, the psychic wound will heal: we will accept our condition and learn to like self and body as it is. We will learn, "It's OK," to be disabled.

It has not worked that way for me. I wanted it to, but it has not. For many years, should someone ask me how I felt about being crippled, I would answer, "It's OK with me! Never think much about it anymore." And indeed this was what I *thought* I believed. But this was just another form of denial at work. It was *not* OK, it has *never* been OK. In fact, I keened over my disability all the time, everyday, all day; I just pretended to myself that I did not.

This was a pretend life and it did not work very well. Now, I do not pretend anymore. I admit my infirmity. I detest it every minute,

I resent having to cart it around with me wherever I go, but I, myself, I *live* in my ghost. If I drive an old, broken-down car, that does not mean that I too am broken down. And my broken-down body is not me. This is, of course, another sort of denial but it is closer to reality. I see it as life affirming.

Disability and denial are inseparable. The reality of disability is unacceptable. I am not this broken-down body; I deny that I am this broken-down body. Yet, bottom line, denial fails and the reality of disability wins. FDR becomes increasingly enfeebled and dies. Mary Pickford grows old and wrinkled and dies. And I too. In my lifelong struggle with disability, I lose. And yet, most paradoxically, somehow, the ghost inside the reality, the self, prevails.

Like Job in the Old Testament, the self does not buckle. It endures the afflictions of disability which, in fact, are no more than the afflictions of Everyman, although earlier and more grievously applied. From this endurance, earlier and more intensely, there comes a kind of Job-like wisdom. In the grand scheme of things—in the great infinite miracle that is life—pain and suffering is trivial. Struggle and crippledness are nothing. What matters is that I am, and it is enough.

In Mitchell's poetic translation[1] of the Hebrew version of the Book of Job, Job's final words to the Unnameable are,

> "I have spoken of the unspeakable
> and tried to grasp the infinite . . .
> I had heard of you with my ears;
> but now my eyes have seen you.
> Therefore I will be quiet,
> comforted that I am dust."

★   ★   ★

This book reflects the maturation of my thought on aspects—personal and public—of being disabled in an able-bodied society. For more than 40 years I have used a wheelchair. For more than 30 years I have been a participant in, and an observer of, the disability revolution. As a writer, I have recorded these observations over the years. The world has changed and so have I.

[1]Mitchell, Stephen, *The Book of Job*, Harperperennial Library, 1992, New York.

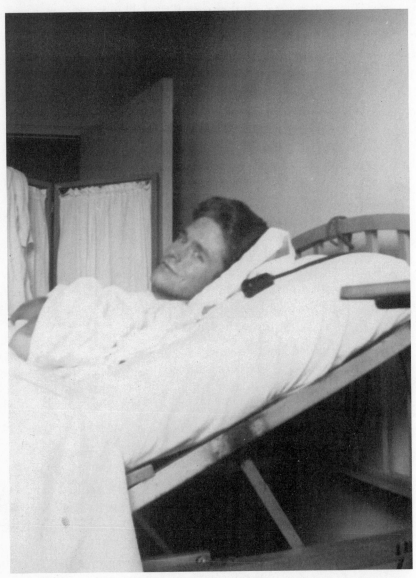

After months of stretching, my body was flexible enough for my head to be elevated. Haircuts in bed were difficult, so I wore my hair long.

THE FIRST SCORE YEARS
CRIPPLED

IT WAS NOT EASY to be a cripple in the society I grew up in.

In 1952 America, disabled people were a hidden minority. There must have been many millions of them, but they were kept out of sight. I was born in 1932. In my first 20 years, I lived in California, Colorado, Chicago, New York City, and Washington, D.C. I attended public schools, always knew my neighborhood by heart, and eagerly explored each new city. Yet today, I can recall having seen only four disabled people over all those years.

When I was about six years old, we lived in Little Neck, a suburb of New York City. I remember there was said to be a "moron" who lived in a house down the block. I think I saw him once— but I may have dreamed it. The shades of that house were always drawn and I was afraid to walk past it. Many years later my mother told me the child had Down's syndrome.

Then there was the popcorn man at Fifth and Main in Grand Junction, Colorado. He was always there at his popcorn stand, seated in his tricycle wheelchair which he operated with curious hand-pedals. I don't know why he was in the wheelchair. We bought popcorn from the man for years, but no one ever knew anything about him.

In Washington, I saw old Senator Capper once, he looked older than any man I had ever seen. He was being pushed onto the Senate floor for a vote. He was in an immense wicker "bath chair" and he appeared to be senile.

Also in Washington, I remember the monkey man who sat on the sidewalk in front of Murphy's Five & Dime on F Street. He was a double amputee at the hips. He had a monkey on a string and he begged for money. It was said that heiress Evelyn Walsh McLean had given him the monkey.

There were of course the Spanish-American War veterans sitting in their wicker wheelchairs on the porch of the Old Soldiers' Home. I would see them on nice days on my way home from school. They did not really count because they were safely interred behind the iron fence of the home.

And that was about it. The disabled were kept out of sight. There were no seriously disabled students in any of the many schools I attended. With certain notable exceptions (e.g., Lionel Barrymore in the Dr. Kildare series), there were no disabled people in the movies. None of my parents' friends were disabled and the disabled were seldom seen on the street.

I did not like the disabled; I was afraid of them. This was something I must have picked up from the people around me. There was, I think, a general, perhaps unconsciously felt, fear of the disabled. This was perhaps not so much a fear of *them* but a fear of what they symbolized—human vulnerability to disease, disability, and death. And people were a great deal more vulnerable back then. Childhood diseases—measles, mumps, whooping cough—were still killers. Scarlet fever and smallpox lurked in recent memory. Influenza and pneumonia, "the old man's friend," were deadly. Malaria and tuberculosis took their toll. Antitoxins and antibiotics were not yet in widespread use, and the famous old family doctor with his black bag could do little more than palliate the suffering. Contagious disease was a legitimate cause for fear.

Disabled people, with their various physical weaknesses, were particularly vulnerable to disease and infection. Pressure sores and gangrene killed many paralytics and amputees; even colds could kill those with weak lungs. The life expectancy of disabled people was not great. Infants with spina bifida, Down's syndrome or other defects were routinely killed at birth to spare them from suffering.

Even if the disabled did live, life was not easy. There was no Medicare, no Medicaid. Most families had no health insurance. There were no Social Security disability payments. The person who was disabled was not expected to work or to live independently. There were, in fact, all sorts of impediments to keep him or her from doing so. Disabled people were expected to live with their families as invalids, "shut-ins." If there was no family support, they lived in public institutions of the sort that housed the insane, the retarded, the paralytic, and lepers. In Grand Junction, Colorado, the institution was out on the edge of town. It was known as "the pest house."

People with disabilities were seen as pests; they were also objects of fun. People with physical deformities were exhibited at freak shows. Midgets and dwarfs were curiosities; they were cooed over or laughed at in travelling shows and vaudeville acts. "Little moron" jokes were all the rage. Comic Jerry Lewis was a great hit with his gibbering imitation of the retarded and his grotesque burlesque of persons with cerebral palsy.

The disabled tended to see themselves as they were seen by others: they were the "sick" member of the family, the shut-in whose life was all but over; no marriage, no career, only a continuing burden to the family. Disabled people lived lives isolated one from another.

The disabled did not see themselves as a community with shared interests or rights. There was no such thing as "disability culture." Most people had never considered that the disabled might have, as a right, access to public facilities such as schools, movies, transportation. Nor had they given thought to the proposition that the disabled should have equal access to employment.

Nevertheless, change was in the air. This change was encouraged by three major developments: the rise of polio epidemics, improved medicine, and the end of World War II.

Polio had become a great human interest story. The epidemics seemed to get worse every year. They struck randomly across the country. The disease was a killer of unknown origin. It struck small children. Those it did not kill, it left with residual paralysis which, with time and care, showed improvement.

Also, polio was highly photogenic. Its effects were visual: little children, wards of patients in iron lungs, wheelchairs and braces. This was important as press photos, photomagazines, and newsreels became important parts of the news business. In the era before television, *Life* magazine showed us each week what was happening and what to think about it.

Franklin Roosevelt was president for more than 12 years, from 1932–1945. He had polio and was, as he said, "a cured cripple." The president founded the March of Dimes and the Polio Foundation, which became the first and most successful of all the private fundraising health agencies.

The foundation launched massive annual fund drives, complete with movie and sports stars and, of course, the active sponsorship of FDR. The press gave it all much attention and as a result virtually everyone in the nation became conscious of the disease and those who had it. There developed an educated, understanding sympathy for the victims of polio.

The first antibiotics were developed during World War II. These, along with sulfa drugs and new therapeutic techniques, gave promise of greatly extending the life expectancy of people with disabilities. This of course raised an important question. Now that a disabled person could look forward to a normal life span, what was he going to do with it?

The first group to benefit from these improvements were the grievously wounded veterans returning from the war. Under the leadership of FDR, plans were made and money allocated for a major rehabilitation effort. With the use of the new medicine, paraplegic veterans survived their wounds. With rehabilitation, they learned how to use the new, compact, and easily maneuverable wheelchairs. With hand controls, they learned to drive their own cars. Using new equipment and techniques, they were able to live on their own, independently.

THE FIRST SCORE YEARS

The Veterans Administration encouraged them to do so, building them one-story houses, giving them new automobiles and generous monthly pensions. This attracted much public attention. There were photo spreads in *Life* and newsreel features. Even a movie, starring Marlon Brando. Americans had an idealist vision of what postwar USA would be like. Everyone would live in the suburbs with a wife and kids, in a Levitt-built house with a car in the garage and a lawn of his own. Now paraplegic veterans were going to share in this future.

Although, in the 1950s, when I contracted polio and the disabled were still being isolated, even warehoused, there was hope that they might be able to live full and healthy lives. More and more, they were doing so. When a disabled person graduated from college or got a job or whatever, it was written up in the newspapers. Increasingly, the disabled were being *seen* and seen to be doing things, having useful lives. The future had begun and, to my surprise, I would be part of it.

POLIO,
MY ACCOUNT

*This is the only detailed account I have ever written of my struggle
with acute polio. I wrote it 20 years after the event. Even after all those
years, it was not easy to write. This piece has been read by only a
handful, and it has never been printed before. I have always thought it
too personal, too painful for publication. Perhaps it will prove helpful
to others as they struggle with their own crises—struggle as Faulkner
put it, not just to endure but to prevail.*

I HAD POLIO in the spring of 1952.

This was an experience now sufficiently rare as to make it worth
recording. The record of the illness is straightforward: the sequence
of events, the physiological happenings, the morbid progress of the
paralysis. This, though, is not the story. It is not the important thing
that was happening. The advancing paralysis, the searing fever, the
body as battleground—these were outward dramas, representative,
but *just* representative, of the inward tragedy taking place. This

involved the collapse of a young man's life, the end of expectation, the passing down of a life sentence without hope of pardon or parole.

It is of this inward experience—to this day to me incredible and inexplicable—that I will try to tell. People survived Dachau and spent the rest of their lives puzzling how. I, too, survived. A young man's life collapsed, but it did not end. My body did not escape its sentence, and I will always be paralyzed. However, my spirit was not paralyzed and never will be. It was stunned, brutalized, raped—too early, too much, grievously. But, as with the Dachau people, it survived. And like them, I do not know how.

The how is what puzzles me and what I hope to reach in this account. To trace the passage of the spirit, it is not enough to say what happened; it is more important to remember, to try to remember, what it *felt* like, to discover what was going on inside as the horrors unfolded without. In general, this should not be a depressing account. The story of a human being learning the fullness of the experience of living, even if the lessons are brutal and quick, is not a sad story. The richness of life and emotions honestly experienced are not sad. My crisis brought with it an emotional clarity and simplicity, a purity of understanding, which altered me forever in ways, 25 years later, I ponder with awe.

It is the desire to share this long search of mine that impels me to try, as so many times before, to record in clear and simple manner what was the central crisis, the central meaning of my life. For within this event, I feel, is the key to everything.

★ ★ ★

I was 19, young and beautiful. I was free. I had broken, to a significant degree, the tight constrictions that bound me to my parents and their cultural values and mores. The discovering and testing of my freedom I found intoxicating. My enthusiasm for sex, for opera, for cars, politics, philosophy, art, and dance was unbounded; the world seemingly lay open before me, mine for the taking. I read, that spring of 1952, the novels of Thomas Wolfe, and Wolfe's appetites were no larger than mine. After a childhood of doing only what was expected, I was at last doing what I wanted.

Against the will of my father in February of that year, I had left the Massachusetts Institute of Technology, a place I hated soundly in every way. Haverford College, a rational, humane, and honest place, had agreed to take me as a student at midyear, and I was happy to go. In my long and checkered career in higher education, no college ever made me happier.

I was intoxicated with life.

I was soon very busy. Classes were small and informal; courses were interesting; assignments were heavy, but not onerous. I bought my first car, a 1940 Ford coupe. The power of the big V-8 engine and the car's lightness gave me a sense of flying, not driving, down the highways. I went into Philadelphia at least once a week for the opera; and for seventy-five cents, I could sit in the top balcony with members of the local Italian community to cheer and boo the favored and not-so-favored tenors. There were concerts and lectures and dates and dancing and, because it was a presidential year, politics.

A lifelong Democrat, I found myself campaigning for Eisenhower during the confusions of the important Pennsylvania presidential primary. I was, of course, strongly for Adlai Stevenson. Governor Stevenson, however, was saying that month that he was not a candidate and would not be a candidate. If, indeed, he did not run, the Democrats would have no attractive candidate. Meanwhile, the Republicans looked as though they were going to nominate Senator Taft, in their usual myopic manner. I felt that '52 would probably be a Republican year and that Taft would be able to beat a weak Democratic candidate. This I considered a catastrophic possibility; hence, I worked hard for the victory of General Eisenhower over Senator Taft. My work consisted mostly of passing out posters for storefronts, posters featuring the General and his famous smile, and riding in an open convertible through the streets of Philadelphia, flanked by hired lovely models adorned with Eisenhower banners, addressing the uninterested populace on the General's merits and throwing Ike buttons at little clumps of people gathered at the bus stops.

It must have been the last weekend in April that a classmate and I drove down to Hood College for a spring weekend. The college weekend—and anyone who has seen the early Debbie Reynolds' movies knows what it was like—was marked by a poignant, important love-making and by my learning how to samba. I became so hot

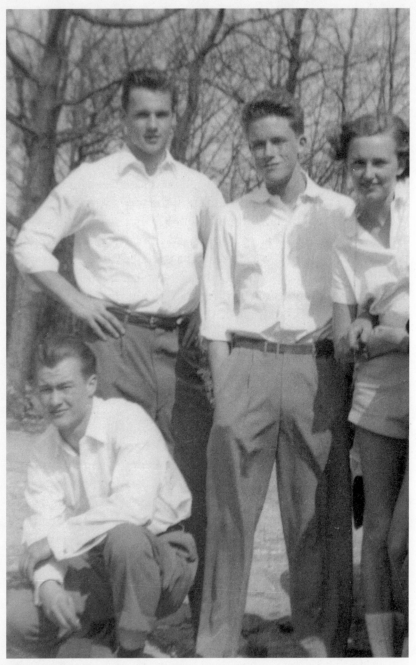

This is the last photo of me taken before I was paralysed by polio. I am standing with Baylis Thomas on my left and Bing Sponsler is kneeling.

and fatigued by the dancing that my girl and I went outside to rest upon the steps of the auditorium in the cool spring evening.

I can remember, even now, the chills I felt: the perspiration of the heat meeting the coolness of the April breezes. This may have been the first physical manifestation of the poliomyelitis virus working within my body. Later that evening, we went and looked through the campus telescope in a tiny observatory and saw the Rings of Saturn. And later still, we made love, my lover and I, for the last time. We did not know it was the last time.

The following week, I came down with a bad cold. This may have slowed my activities, but it did not stop them, for I was young and I was strong.

The next weekend, Haverford College sent a delegation to a mock political convention at Harrisburg. The Haverford delegation—and I was an enthusiastic member—was pledged to the drafting of Adlai Stevenson, protests or no. In a long night's work on the convention floor, we pulled it off. With what was close to a genuine, spontaneous draft, the delegates in the hall came around to our enthusiasm, and the Governor was nominated. We sent him a wire of notification and congratulations, a wire, which I am certain, he acknowledged in some graceful manner. During the weekend, I developed laryngitis, a chronic complaint, and a severe sore throat. I was becoming acutely uncomfortable.

April that year was lovely—warm and promising. Many an afternoon I spent on the lawn in the walled library garden, reading my Thomas Wolfe novels in the sun. Many an evening I spent studying to the strains of *La Traviata*, the windows open to the spring night.

In retrospect, I was the young Thomas Wolfe, spreading wide my arms to encompass the experience, the emotion, all the world has to offer. In retrospect, the love of Violetta and Alfredo in their beautiful duet was my love for a life just beginning.

The college faced Lancaster Pike, which was the beginning of Highway 30, the Lincoln Highway. It stretched from Philadelphia to the West Coast, passing through such places as Cheyenne, Laramie, and Rawlins, Wyoming. Late at night, I would yearn for the West. Why not, I would think, why not go down to the college gate and start hitchhiking tonight and be in Wyoming by the end of the week? The

West had a strong and permanent call for me. And yet, the farthest west I was to get that weekend was a mile and a half down the pike to Bryn Mawr Hospital.

Upon our return from Harrisburg, serious things began to happen to my physical state. I developed a backache that was annoying and painful, and my neck was unaccountably stiff. I went to the school nurse with my pains. She did not take my temperature, nor anything else, but, listening to my complaints, blamed them on my lying on the wet and dewy grass and gave me aspirin tablets for my discomfort.

Wednesday, the pain increased, and Wednesday night, I had no sleep. My roommate, a premed student, slept in the bottom of our double bunk bed, and he complained that my tossing kept him awake and annoyed him throughout the night. He called me a hypochondriac.

The next day, the pain continued. That night, I made no attempt whatever to sleep in bed. It was agony for me to lie down; it was agony to sit in an armchair, and every step sent shudders of pain through my legs, up and down my spine, the whole length of my body. I spent the night in the showers, with water as hot as I could stand pouring down my back. The warmth brought some surcease from pain; come morning, I returned to the school's infirmary. The nurse again gave me aspirins and admonitions. She did, however, urge that I come back to see the doctor, who would be at the infirmary in the afternoon.

I spent the morning attempting to register for the courses I would be taking in the fall. This preregistration required moving about the campus from professor to professor and, naturally enough, required climbing stairs. I found this quite difficult; my legs tired quickly and the pain of that, and the jarring pain from each footstep, had, if anything, increased.

A friend of mine, who himself had had polio several years before, actually believed that I was coming down with the disease. He was beside himself. He did not wish to scare me, but—and for this I will always be grateful to him—he insisted that I return to my room and that I let him take over my preregistration chores. Later, I learned that he was so disturbed by what was happening to me that he went home that evening to tell his parents of his fears.

I did see the doctor that afternoon. He was a kindly older man, who told me I was quite ill and that I did, indeed, have a temperature.

He urged that I go into the infirmary at once. This, I assured him, was quite impossible. My parents were arriving that evening from Washington for Parents' Weekend, and I must be on hand to welcome them. I promised, however, that after I had welcomed them, I would then turn myself over to the infirmary.

What I told the doctor was quite true, but it was by no means the whole truth. I was in extreme tension. Nothing remotely as serious as this had ever happened to my body. Something was very, very wrong—and getting worse, hour by hour. I could not admit to the doctor how serious, how wrong this was, because I would not even begin to admit it to myself. The admission would have caused hysterical fears of a size I had never experienced. I had no conscious experience with large emotions. I had been trained through years to suppress them all. Emotions of any sort were not allowed to show in my family. The fear that my illness was causing, the fear threatening to burst through all repressions, was as alarming to me as the illness itself.

Coming down the steps from the dining hall that night, my right knee buckled. I caught myself and did not lose my balance. It was the first sign of paralysis.

It must have been about nine o'clock in the evening when my parents arrived. I was sitting on the couch in my room in the dormitory when my father came in the door. I rose to greet him, and my knee buckled again. Again, I did not fall. This time, I braced my leg quickly with my arm. I do not believe that my father noticed. I went out to the car to greet my mother and sister.

At the car, I told them that I was not feeling well. I intended to spend the night in the infirmary, but I was certain that by tomorrow I would be well enough to give them a tour of the college and the Main Line communities. I wanted so much for them to appreciate Haverford and to respect my judgment in leaving M.I.T. for this small liberal arts college. The weekend was to be a reconciliation. They would understand and give their approval at last to my new life.

And as I recall the moment, there is an ache that will not go away at the innocence of us all. My parents seemed so young, so inexperienced, so unaware. They had led star-blessed lives; neither of them had known sickness, pain, or adversity. Mother had been always beautiful and popular; father was most likely to succeed. Theirs had been a childhood romance, a marriage without surface flaw, and with friends, children, and success. They had not suffered because, indeed, their lives had been lived upon the very surface of things, without the deep joys and sorrows of fully-felt emotions and experience.

Already, throughout my growing up, I had learned to hide the deep and passionate angers that I felt, to dampen the highs of my joys, as well as the depths of my feelings when talking with them; for they were, throughout their lives, true innocents.

I feel sometimes that I was born sad. From childhood, I had always heard "the eternal note of sadness" of Matthew Arnold's *Dover Beach*. And so, I feel the ache of innocence and the sadness of parting when I relive that evening in early May.

With my father, I went down the six steps of the dormitory to the car at the curb. I told my waiting mother and sister that I was ill and should go to the infirmary for the night. In response to the rather searching questions of my mother, I replied that I did not know what was wrong, that I was in some pain, but that, undoubtedly, I would be well enough in the morning to show them around the campus.

Mother said, when she heard that my neck and back were sore, "Oh, dear, I hope you do not have polio." I remember assuring her that she was being silly; it was not even the polio season, after all. I said I would be well enough in the morning to show them about the campus, and I was not lying: I was counting on a miracle. At that stage of pain and fatigue—I had not slept for 48 hours—nothing short of a miracle would bring relief.

I refused their gentle offer that they drive me to the infirmary; and so, my family—my mother, my father, my sister, and my dog, which they had brought with them—walked with me across the old and quiet campus from my dormitory to the infirmary. I asked that we walk on the grass as the pavement caused jarring steps, which made walking even more painful to me.

We walked together across the campus; it was my last walk. I will never walk again.

This was the last of many foolish things I had done concerning my sickness. Later, in research on poliomyelitis, I found that the sooner the patient takes to his bed, the less likely it is his paralysis will be extensive or severe. My refusal to stop my activities, even as my legs were buckling, greatly increased the possibility of permanent paralysis. Polio, however, is so erratic and unpredictable in its paralytic patterns that, in any given case, it is probably nonsense to say because of this, that happened.

It must have been about 9:30 that night when we entered the infirmary. I had a small room, crisp sheets on the bed, a gray-haired nurse in a starched clean uniform. There was, I remember, a little bedside lamp, which cast a warm and comforting light. The room opened directly onto the lobby of the small building and was separated from it by a pair of glass French doors, which had sheer gauze-like curtains to ensure privacy. The shadowy outlines of persons standing in the lobby were thrown upon the curtains in silhouette.

I went promptly to bed. I was too fatigued to sit up; and by then, the pain was so great that position made little difference. The agony was total.

I was learning an important lesson; there is a point with pain beyond which there can be no increased intensity. It is, perhaps, like hysteria: once you are truly hysterical, that's it. You do not, you cannot, become more and more hysteric. Total pain consumes the body, consumes the senses, consumes the intellect, but it is bearable. The *fear* of pain is intolerable, but pain itself is bearable. Ultimately, as I was to learn well, it is a very simple matter: pain will be endured until the point at which it can no longer be endured, and then you pass out. If the pain continues intensely enough, for long enough, you die. That is all there is to pain. These are very simple verities—life becomes very simple in the presence of total pain.

I went quietly to bed and listened to father discuss my case with the nurse in the lobby outside the room. I watched their shadows on the curtains of the door. My father told the nurse that he and mother had always been concerned about the possibility of polio and that they would appreciate her calling a doctor. The nurse still comforted herself with the hope that my problem was a chill. I had no wish to see a doctor for fear he would detect how very sick I was. My pain was intense, and my temperature was mounting at a notable rate. Reluctantly, I sided with my father, and a doctor was called.

The doctor came, finally—the kindly doctor who had seen me in the afternoon. He did various things, tapping my knees, my elbows, using a stethoscope, taking my pulse. He listened to my story. By then, I was not hysteric, I was in despair. I had never taken drugs. I had never had a sleeping pill in my life. I knew nothing of painkillers. I had no idea whether he could help me or not. I told the doctor as forcefully as I could that my agony had become unbearable. I told him, as I had not told him in the afternoon, that I had been two nights without sleep. As I talked, I let slip—I, at last, let all my symptoms slip. I told the truth and gave him a full account of the frightening, gradual, yet ineluctable thing that had come upon my body.

I begged him for something, anything, to help with the pain. He was, as I have said, most comforting, and he said that what I needed was a good night's sleep. That seemed so bland and meager an assessment of my needs that I had trouble keeping back my tears. As the doctor talked, he brought out from his bag a small vial of pills and rolled into the palm of his hand a single, minuscule white tablet. He assured me this would do the trick. I took the tablet, but could not believe that anything that small could in any significant way assuage my pain. But I was wrong; it was pure morphine. The pain receded from my consciousness as tide from a beach, smoothly and imperceptibly. I slept with the honesty of a baby, untroubled by pain or dream. It was an astonishing business.

I awoke in the middle of the night with a strong desire to urinate. In getting out of bed, I found that my legs had, unaccountably, turned into something like stiff rubber. The knee joints would not hold. Sitting on the edge of the bed, very carefully I straightened each leg, and, by leaning over and placing my hands firmly upon the kneecaps, I was able to stabilize my legs sufficiently so that I could walk to the bathroom. There, I noticed another peculiar thing: I could not urinate. I had a strong desire to do so. There was obviously a good deal of urine in my bladder, but it would not come out. This seemed strange, but I was heavily doped by morphine, and so I went back to bed where I promptly went to sleep again. Those were the last steps I will ever take in this world. There should have been more ceremony attached to them.

I awoke at something like six in the morning. The spring sunlight filled the room with lightness and shown across the bed. It was a glorious spring morning. I felt splendid, and I savored the fresh air, the sunlight, and the sense of well-being—for the morphine had not yet worn off. However, it was even then in the process of doing so. The pain was coming back with a grim relentless insistence.

Sleep had done me good, and by comparison, even with the increasing pain, I felt much better than I had the night before. The nurse had insisted that I call her upon waking in the morning, but I chose to put this off for a bit and to lie in my bed in the bright early morning sunlight and think about all that was happening.

I had been a fat, helpless little boy, who had detested his body and its failures. During my adolescent years with diet and exercise, I had changed my body from a soft and yielding thing into a trim, solid, responsive figure. I was proud of my work; my achievement had given me substantial self-confidence. I believed, and there was no reason to doubt it, that I was in condition to go anywhere, to do anything. In fact, that very summer, I was scheduled to sail as a member of an Arctic expedition, which intended to go overland by dog sled to the North Pole. I was certain I had the endurance for such a feat, and I looked forward to it. It seemed unthinkable that this body of mine should fall prey to major sickness. As the fat and pasty boy, I had all the childhood diseases and numerous psychosomatic complaints as well. But that had been a period of my life now far behind me. I had not liked myself as that fat and pasty boy, and I had, as it were, rebuilt the material; I was now the new model. I was young, strong, and invincible. Disease did not enter into my plans. But, of course, disease was at that very moment entering into my life.

As I lay thinking, the actual paralyzing process began, first with the toes of my left leg. I am not sure now how I came to notice that the toes of my left foot would no longer wiggle. Somehow, I was just aware of the matter. I could send the usual message, in the usual way, from my will to my foot—"move"—but there was no movement. It was an interesting phenomenon and puzzling business. I experimented with each toe to determine how extensive was the lack of movement. Even as I experimented, the lack of movement seemed to expand its area. Soon, in a matter of minutes, the foot and ankle were powerless. There was no loss of sensation—in fact, just the reverse. The sensory nerves of my body—throughout my body—were inflamed. I did not for an instant believe that the paralysis was permanent or caused by poliomyelitis because I had always assumed that a paralyzed limb would be senseless as well, and my limbs were hypersensitive.

The paralysis gradually worked its way up my left leg. I remember sliding my right foot and ankle under my left and using the motor power of my right leg to move my inert left leg back and forth across the bed. As I say, it was a strange business. Once the paralysis had worked its way up to my left hip, it seemed to stop. I half expected that it would momentarily go away—as though the leg had simply "fallen asleep" for a second or two. The whole paralytic process had taken not much more than half an hour. Now, I expected it—perhaps still hoping for miracles—to reverse itself and work its way back down the leg. It did not do so.

I called the nurse and told her about this strangeness. She remained very calm within the room; but, calling the doctor from the lobby, she was anything but calm. He told her to send for an ambulance and that he would meet me at the hospital. He then called my parents at their hotel in downtown Philadelphia. My sister told me years later that, on the drive from the hotel to the hospital, no one said a word. Each of the three was certain that I had polio, yet each was determined not to alarm the other two by speaking of it.

By the time the ambulance arrived, the paralysis was working its way *down* my right leg. It had come up the left and was now going down the right. By the time I was in the ambulance, both legs were completely paralyzed.

As the ambulance man came into the room, I began to live, as it were, on two levels. This continued, as I remember, for at least the next two or three weeks. At the here and now level, I was in great agony and terribly sick. On the other level, I was an observer to the disaster. I was watching the events from outside my body, outside my life, as though suspended above it all. And as over the next several days, my condition worsened, the distance of this, my other self, from my body seemed to lengthen until, at one point, the grave problems overwhelming my physical body seemed to be very small and very far away, indeed.

Curious details remain in the memory. I remember the infirmary nurse as a white-haired, crotchety, but essentially motherly woman, who, in the many years she had watched over Haverford infirmary, had never before had a serious case of anything to nurse. I remember when the ambulance men came into the room, I was concerned less they feel uneasy: I was embarrassed about my inability to walk. I tried to make light of my condition, to be cheerful and helpful. The ambulance stretcher could not get through the narrow hallway to my bedroom, and it was necessary to be placed in a canvas bag-type carrier. Now, as I think about it, it seems likely they used one of those bags with which bodies are carted away to the morgue. This is how I feel about the matter, now. As I was being carried out the front door of the infirmary, I met two of my classmates coming in. It was very early for them to be going to the infirmary; perhaps they were ill. I waved to them brightly as we passed. I urged the ambulance men to use the siren on the way to the hospital, which they did. I always ask them to use the siren when I am riding in an ambulance.

There were a lot of people coming in and out. I had been taken to the contagious ward and placed in a private room. The ward was housed in a shabby, little one-story wood frame building constructed during some war or other for some epidemic. It was connected to the main hospital buildings by means of a covered walkway. The people coming in and out of my room wore surgical masks. I did not find this strange, but then, I had never been in a hospital before. It certainly did not occur to me that I had something that might be contagious or that I was in some medical way unclean, dangerous.

Once the paralysis was evident, I was taken off all painkillers. Analgesics, from aspirin to morphine, deaden pain by acting upon the central nervous system. Polio is a disease of the central nervous system, and when such things of life-giving importance as the breathing response are inhibited, as by paralytic polio, the analgesic serves to assist the disease in deadening the response. Throughout the crisis, I was without painkillers; and, thus, I was always fully conscious and fully sensitive to all that was happening.

The doctors—for now there were far more than one doctor, there were many—could not at first, and would not later, tell me the cause of my distress. "A form of neuritis," they said; that is, an inflammation of the nervous system. It would take a variety of tests to arrive at a definitive diagnosis, they said. In any case, the illness was severe, and recuperation would not be quick. Even though I was told this, and even though I understood what I had been told, I repeatedly sought reassurance that I would be released by Monday, so that I could finish a term paper due the middle of the following week. In such way does the mind cling rigorously to small habits and duties in the face of major calamity.

Major calamities are hard to comprehend. The mind will not accept at once the overnight disintegration of a lifetime's work, the permanence of a paralysis. The mind does not know how to cope with finalities of such scale and size; it continues to deal with the daily and mundane: the term paper due on Monday, the dance on Saturday night. Only slowly does the horror seep in.

For me, over the first days, there was no sense whatsoever of permanent alterations being made. In fact, in those days, no one knew—certainly not the doctors—how lasting, extensive, or severe the paralysis might be. And there was in truth little time for thoughtful contemplation of what was occurring. I was in crisis, and, as I remember, my entire concentration, the concentration of both mind and body, was devoted to the struggle with the disease. The struggle was intense, exhausting, and constant. It is important to emphasize how intellectually and emotionally demanding disease is. Like a military campaign, it demands time, energy, planning, strategy, cleverness, and luck. It fills the day.

I was placed on a standard hospital mattress, which, now that the morphine had worn off, I found intolerably painful. After searching the hospital, a new sponge rubber mattress was found, and I was transferred to it. I was pulled from the old mattress onto the new by means of a draw-sheet, a simple enough procedure. In my case, it was not so simple. Any jar, touch, or shift in my body position produced new pain. In order to pull me across the one bed to the other, without unduly disturbing my position, it was necessary to have several people at each side of the draw-sheet. In those days, polio was rightly

feared and wrongly believed to be contagious. Volunteers were necessary to assist the nurses moving me, and several of the janitorial
staff volunteered; they were courageous to do so. Even wearing caps,
gowns, and surgical masks, they were exposing themselves, and perhaps their children, to a dreaded possibility. I am grateful to them;
and, today, 25 years later, I can remember their faces, if not their
names.

Doctors, residents, and interns were in and out. Tests of all sorts
were performed. Only one spinal tap was taken. I believe that a tap
without anesthetic, can be a very painful business. The one performed on me without anesthetic was irrelevant. My central nervous system could produce no more pain than it was already sending
out. I can remember the variation and levels of intensity caused during the test by the necessity of turning me on my side and rearrang-
ing my legs; I can remember no particular novel or heightened degree
of pain as a result of the spinal tap needle itself.

For some reason, perhaps based on misguided kindness, the doctors refused to tell me my diagnosis, other than to say, as they had
been saying, that I had contracted some form of virulent neuritis. As
the doctors had successfully dodged my direct questions, I decided to
probe indirectly. And so, when a new face, a resident I had not seen
before, came in to examine me, I asked him just how bad a case of
polio I had. He replied, "We do not know yet. We will just have to wait
and see how it develops." When my parents came to see me later in
the day, I told them I had polio; and they replied, "Yes, we know." This
confirmed to me what the resident had said, as it were, *en passant*.

By that time, I was very busy with the struggle against the disease,
and I had little strength of intellect left to ponder the meaning of
this diagnosis. As a child, my family had moved often; and I, of
course, went with them. It seemed we moved from polio epidemic
to polio epidemic; polio had been an every summer occurrence. I disliked the disease because swimming pools were always shut during an
epidemic: it was believed polio was transmitted through the pool
water. Remember this was before air conditioning and swimming
pools were virtually the only form of relief from the heat. Thus, my
only contact with the disease had been the discomfort caused by the
loss of my daily swim. None of my friends had ever contracted polio.

I had seen the short, filmed appeals of Sister Kenny and the March of Dimes, which were shown in local movie houses. On the silver screen, there would appear a picture of Kenny gently lifting and lowering the little leg of a smiling child in a physical therapy exercise. Give to the March of Dimes, Greer Garson or some other movie star would say. The houselights would then come up, and the ushers would pass through the theater, collecting contributions, passing the contribution can up one aisle and down the next, like a collection plate in church.

I remember the child was smiling. I had no knowledge that polio hurt terribly; I had no knowledge that the limbs would stiffen, the joints freeze with adhesions. I believed paralysis meant the loss of sensory as well as motor abilities, and I had no idea whether the paralysis was permanent or not.

I had always disliked the handicapped very much. I would cross the street, rather than pass by a severely handicapped person. I remember, during one March of Dimes fund drive, there was an iron lung on display in front of the Capitol Theater. It made me feel uncomfortable, and I crossed the street to avoid passing by it.

I abhorred illness and despised personal weakness. I insisted with a martial discipline that my body serve as I directed. I was handsome; I would be lean, strong, and tireless. In the naive day of my youth, I believed this possible and, so far, it had been. Suddenly, of course, it was no longer possible. I had been overwhelmed by disease, sandbagged by fate. The diagnosis of paralytic polio carried with it, by implication, a life sentence of disability. This should have been the subject of very great concern to me, but it was not. Not then. Later, much later, much later still, the concern would become engulfing. Then, it was the onrush of the disease itself which commanded all my skills and perceptions.

Polio was a battleground, no less dangerous than any war. The battleground was within me; the struggle was waged, the life-or-death decisions were made, within me. Nurses, doctors, family actually played little part in the battle itself. They supplied, or not, the weapons and supports I needed. Whatever struggles were going on within them, whatever prayers or devotions or attention they lavished upon me, the action was all mine, internal.

I do not remember food, nor do I remember taking water, although surely with my high temperature and resultant dehydration, I must have done so. I remember being catheterized. A young intern stuck a rubber tube, about the size of a soda straw, up through the urethra of my penis and thereby drained my bladder. Later, a permanent catheter was inserted, which had a small deflated balloon attached to its end. Once the catheter was in place, the balloon was inflated in my bladder, thus keeping the catheter from slipping out. The catheter was attached by a rubber tubing to a bottle under the bed, and my bladder was free to drain at will. This arrangement worked well, although, in time, infections would occur. Nothing whatever was done about my bowels; the movement of my limbs and body were too painful to attempt any sort of evacuation. For some two weeks, I lay upon my back, immobile.

On Saturday, the day I entered the hospital, the paralysis seemed to have ceased its advance. Both legs were paralyzed; the muscles of my trunk were weakened, but still functioning. My arms and neck, lungs, and the muscles of the upper body generally were functioning well. My temperature, however, remained high. I believe it was in the range of 105 degrees. On Sunday, the trunk muscles weakened further; and, as the day progressed, my arms became weak and my breathing became labored. By evening, an oxygen tent was placed over me. This produced a blessed, although temporary, relief. The oxygen, I remember, smelled as pure, as clear and life-giving, as the air at timberline of the mountains of Colorado. This sense of life and memory of Colorado sustained me for hours. I did not sleep through the night, but I dozed with daydream-like visions of my beloved Colorado.

By early Monday morning, my arms and hands were paralyzed; my neck was paralyzed. I was finding it difficult, and soon impossible, to swallow. My eyes ceased to function normally; I developed double, triple, quadruple, erratic vision, and, most important of all, the oxygen seemed to be running out. I remember complaining to the nurses that the tank must be empty, for I could find no refreshment or sustenance from the air within the oxygen tent. The nurses, for there were two, assured me the tank was full, the tent was functioning. I lay there, concentrating upon each breath. Each breath became a conscious decision, an exhausting labor, less and less satisfying, ever more tiring.

Upon consideration, it seemed strange that I was not then more desperate about my condition. Totally paralyzed, fighting for breath, with no further assistance expected or conceived of, why was I not in a state of panic and fear? The answer must be that I was too busy. The intense concentration required by breathing left no time for philosophical pondering or emotional excesses. Trapped in a burning building, all one's skills, both physical and mental, are devoted to survival. Not until afterwards come the shock, the hysterics, the collapse.

It must have been around noon on Monday that I was operated on. Unbeknownst to me, a doctor, expert in the functioning of the lungs, had been placed on 24-hour alert. As my breathing began to fail rapidly, the doctor was summoned from central Philadelphia. He was brought to Bryn Mawr Hospital by motorcycle police escort, sirens screaming—a sight I would love to have seen. I was told that he was on the way, and that he would be able to help my breathing. I was not told how, but the hope became conviction; and my efforts now had a target—to hold out until he arrived.

No one warned me that surgery was to be performed, although, in fact, the doctor had come to perform a tracheotomy. This is a simple procedure; a cut is made through the trachea below the vocal cords and a silver breathing tube three inches long is inserted into the trachea. It extends directly to the lungs. By attaching a line from an oxygen tank directly to the trachea tube, the lungs are supplied with fresh oxygen without passing through the rather long passages of the nostrils and trachea clogged with fluids. The trachea tube also makes it possible to evacuate fluids from the lungs by means of a nasty-sounding, nasty-feeling, little rubber hose vacuum cleaner. This is called aspiration.

I was much too sick to be moved to a surgery theater, and so, the operation was performed at bedside. I remember it well. As I was too sick to be moved, so, too, was I too sick for anesthetics. There was not time to explain the procedure to be followed, nor its purpose. No explanation was given me as to the benefits of the operation or the effects I would feel, once my trachea was opened. Very bright and hot lights were brought into the room, and my memory is one of dazzling brilliance. Although my eyesight was by then most peculiar, I was still able to see.

The doctor wore glasses. He worked feverishly and held his head close to his work. This meant that his eyeglasses served as a mirror for me. In the bright light, clearly reflected, I could watch his hand as he slit my throat. As he inserted the tube, there was a slight rush of air into my lungs. This was followed by nothing: a very strong sense of nothingness, a finality. My nose and my mouth, struggling to gulp air and force it into my lungs, suddenly were left gasping. They were impotent at last. I had an acute and overwhelming sense of suffocation, as my mouth and nostrils were now powerless to assist in obtaining air. I tried desperately to tell the doctor my concern. I felt that he had made some ghastly mistake, that, inadvertently, he had blocked off my access to the small amount of air I was still able to breathe. The doctor who knew that, indeed, I would suffocate presently unless I was placed in an iron lung at once did not have time, did not take time, to explain to me that air was entering my lungs through the tube in my trachea, contrary to whatever feelings were being experienced by my mouth and nostrils. I was in an extreme state of panic.

Standing by were the volunteers who had assisted in transferring mattresses. Now, they stepped forward, shoulder to shoulder, each placing his forearms under me. Then, lifting together, they clasped me to their collective bosom and ran—I remember them running—they ran with me out of the room, down the hall to the room where the iron respirator was waiting.

An iron lung of the 1950's vintage was a large machine, some seven feet long, shaped like a large tin can. At one end was an electrically-operated bellows, and at the other, a neckpiece. The patient was placed on a pallet inside the lung; the lid was shut, and the patient's head stuck out through the neckpiece. The bellows would pump away, night and day, pulling air into the can and then forcing it out. The vacuum this created would cause the patient's lungs to expand and contract, and life would be sustained, as long as the pumping continued. The machine, so important, so truly traumatic, was simplicity itself.

My last memory is of being laid out on the pallet and inserted into the tin can of the iron lung. At this point, I passed out from suffocation because of the paralysis of my respiratory muscles.

The machine was turned on, and the machine revived me.

I regained consciousness, a prisoner of the iron lung. Flat on my back, I was unable to see my body because it was within the machine. Only my head, stuck through a sponge rubber collar, was outside the can and in the world. Without a pillow for my head, my eyes stared straight upwards where, mounted to the lung, there was a mirror at a 45-degree angle. This became my mirror on the outside world. Everything I was to see over the next six weeks, I saw through this mirror. People, while talking to me, would look at the mirror if they wished to make eye contact.

There are prisoners in small and windowless prison cells, but they usually have a small grillwork in their cell door. Through this, they are able to look directly at their corridor, at their jailer, man to man, eye to eye. With their vision, they may roam their cells, which has become their world, inspecting minutely the details of the floor, the walls, the fixtures; they retain proprietary ownership of their bodies. They are able to clean, care, and pleasure themselves; the iron lung patient has no such freedoms. His world is his field of vision, and this is dictated by the mirror and its angle and the direction in which the lung is placed.

My temperature at its highest point was, I believe, 108 degrees. I was never delirious but conscious. I did not sleep, but lived for days in a strange state of semi-awareness and conscious daydreaming. It was during this period that my sense of separability was at its greatest. On the "real" level, I was conscious, struggling against the disease, fighting off fatigue, maintaining contact and communication with nurses, doctors. Throughout, I was cheerful, optimistic, helpful. On the other level, I was present, all right; I was in the room, watching all that was going on, but I was somehow removed.

I asked for last rites, and they were given me. The request was surprising. I had not been aware that religion was an important or significant matter to me, though I had for several years made a show of piety and devotion. Whether the request was genuinely felt or simply a theatrical gesture, I do not know. Whether the sacrament received gave comfort, I do not remember. It is my impression that it did.

My father tells me that the doctors asked him for permission to perform an autopsy on me after my death. He refused to believe that I would die and would not discuss the matter with them. This request became my father's principal memory of those days; it was his most keenly felt experience. To me, the request, or even the fact of autopsy, seems of minuscule importance. How different are we, my father and I. Upon what different levels of experience and perception do human beings operate?

My sister remembers that, during the operation, my parents and she were huddled in a corner of the hospital lobby. She says the doctor came from my bed to them, my fresh blood splattered across his surplice. It spurted when he had cut open my throat. He told them medicine had done all that it could; there was nothing more to be done. She says that, for reasons she does not remember, they seem to have spent the rest of the day seated in the family car. It was raining, and they were crying.

So, what was all this like? What was it like, after the last rites had been said, totally paralyzed, unable to breathe, unable to swallow, sight distorted, the sense of smell and taste gone crazy, nothing in the body responding to direction from motor, sensory, or autonomic nervous systems? With all but a very few nerve cells dead or dying, what was it like?

Life in death, death in life? Life/death? I think that it was this question and my answer to it that filled the two weeks of crisis. Although never phrased as succinctly, as starkly, the question was certainly the issue on which my mind focused. For I was convinced then, as I am convinced now, that the question was a real one and that, for at least two weeks, I had the freedom—or perhaps the responsibility—to choose one or the other. I could live or I could die, and for two weeks, I stalled my decision. I delayed my answer.

Throughout life, there is always the spectre of death; suicide is always an alternative. Suicide, however, requires not only the decision, but the action itself; it is necessary to take one's life by a positive act. During the two-week crisis of my disease, the matter was simpler. It required no "action" on my part to die. It was no longer necessary to move from the state of living to the state of death. The move had already been made by the disease—the avenue was there; all that was required was the decision to take it. As the fever raged and the virus was at its work destroying my central nervous system, nothing further was required of me—no slicing of wrists, no gulping of pills. All that was required was a change of attitude; I could let go. Let go, cease the struggle—and the pain, the hurt, the fatigue, the effort would be over. It was, as it remains, very tempting.

This may give the impression that I lay on my pallet in the iron lung for two weeks, working in some sort of philosophical manner on the resolution of an existential dialectic. This, of course, was far from true. There was, in fact, very little time for musing. I was busy. As I have said, being very sick takes one's time and attention. I and my nurses, for I had two private duty nurses a shift, were very busy. At times, they were frantic. It is surprising how much work is involved in maintaining blood transfusions, glucose intravenous feedings, oxygen supply, catheterization, ice packs, hot packs, the endless adjustments to the body and the equipment—needs that followed one another throughout the day and night.

I was aware of no great sense of drama; the atmosphere was rather more like the La Guardia air flight control tower on a Friday evening. It was a sense of intense concentration and high competence. The nurses knew what they must do; I learned, for my body told me, what I must do—that is, what I must do *if* I chose to survive.

At that time, I felt no sense of loss. I was not then aware that the paralysis—some, or perhaps all of it—would be permanent. The idea of life with a substantially altered body, with a body that functioned other than it had always functioned, was unknown to me; it was a thought then unthinkable because I had never thought it. In the same manner, being seriously ill had always been unthinkable to me; and, yet, here I was, ill beyond all comprehension. The fact that I, Hugh Gallagher, was terribly ill was a concept that took me a long time to comprehend. That the price of survival was permanent and severe paralysis has taken me many years to comprehend. Had I, in fact, understood the price of survival, as I now understand it, I am not at all clear that my decision would have been, as it was, to live.

My decision was certainly not an informed one. It was the result of a medical conspiracy, and I was the victim of a swindle. The conspiracy had as participants my family, the doctors and nurses, and, I suppose, the values of society. They are not my values. Never, at any time during the crisis, was I told what my body could reasonably be expected to be like after having been savaged by the disease; never was there the slightest indication of what the battlefield would be like after the war. "We made a desert and called it Victory," said the Roman senator of Carthage. The doctors could well have said the same of me. Victory was their strategy and, without consultation or consent, they used every weapon available to them.

For weeks, my life was maintained by artificial means. Without those means, I would have died instantly, effortlessly. Throughout the crisis, every effort was made to sustain life, without a single thought being given to the *quality* of the life once it had been sustained.

This was a quarter of a century ago before the extraordinary developments in life support machinery. The situation I faced then was a rare one; now, it is all too common. Do doctors, does the medical profession, have an ethical right to commandeer that most basic and private decision—whether to live or die? I think not. There is, indeed, a time to live and a time to die, and this should be principally a matter for a man himself to decide. The medical profession should be available to help the patient, to provide him an appraisal of his situation, to advise him of his rights as in the legal profession. But they should not attempt to make the decision for him in some mindless obsession with the preservation of life at any price, no matter how grotesque the results. Life itself is not a value higher than the dignity and integrity of the self, the freedom of the will.

Jefferson's "The price of liberty is eternal vigilance," speaks not just of tyrants, but of doctors.

I was never once asked whether I wished to receive yet another life support assist. The doctors with their devices were in treacherous combat with the disease; and I just happened to be the site of battle. At no time was I acknowledged, in the sense that I was consulted or included in the strategy devised by the doctors. I was simple "patient material," and my presence was accidental.

And so, there were two games in town: the doctors whacking away at the disease with the insane gusto of medieval surgeons, and my own studied assessment of whether to live or to die. Without the doctors, I would not have had the option, true. But had I decided to give up, their game—with all its machines—would have been over and done, period.

This is, of course, retrospective judgment. I did not protest. It is just foolish to attempt a description of my situation. I was not doped; I was not sedated. I was not tranquilized; I was in full, indeed, overpowering awareness of my senses, and what I sensed was pain.

As there is a threshold of pain, so there is an upper limit beyond which the body cannot register. A stereo system can go so loud; an engine can generate so many horsepower; the body can feel only so much pain. Go beyond that, inflict twice as much punishment, and the body will not be able to experience twice as much pain. Variations and combinations of pain are possible: virtually unlimited changes may be rung, but the sum of pain experienced cannot exceed the boundary. The outer limit has been reached. Pain is like death; there is just so much, and that's it. Megadeaths have no meaning.

I lived for at least two weeks at the outer limits of pain. I was, however, well trained to hide my emotions. As a child, I had not been encouraged to express my feelings or, indeed, allowed to admit to having them. And so in the hospital I knew what was expected of me. With but few exceptions, I lived up to these expectations. I was of good cheer; I was a good sport; I complained as little as possible. I was helpful and cooperative, encouraging and inquisitive, aware and thoughtful at all times of the feelings of others. I was, in fact, the person I had been trained since infancy to be. For so many years I had worn a mask, I was not, even at this moment, aware that it was a mask. As my life was collapsing, as my body was turning from muscle to water, and the cells upon which health and movement depended were dying by the millions, I remained a well-brought-up, courteous and considerate, upper middle-class child.

And as the mask was impenetrable, as the wall was unscalable, there was no way for me to reach out for comfort and support, no way to share or have acknowledged the deep terror of the unknown, the agony of pain. I could not reach out, and I knew no way of letting in those who would help, those who would share, those who would acknowledge and give comfort and support. Whatever I must bear, I must bear alone. Whatever was happening to me, whatever my feelings were, however desperately I yearned for help and understanding in the face of these terrible things—none of this was reflected upon my expression or my demeanor. I was, I believe, a perfect patient.

This memory of emotional isolation fills me today with a terror far exceeding the fears aroused by a recounting of the physiological events of my disease. It is conceivable I could live through similar events again; it is inconceivable that I would be able to do so alone, masking my emotions, denying my needs.

I regained consciousness and entered into a new routine of living. The iron lung in its clumsy manner did its breathing for me. I was breathing pure oxygen through a tube inserted into my tracheotomy. Every hour or so, my lungs were aspirated—a rubber hose suction device was stuck down the tracheotomy tube into my lungs, and the fluids were removed, which, if left in place, would promptly have caused pneumonia and death by drowning. When it became necessary to nurse my body, a large heavy clear plastic hemisphere was clamped over my head—as a deep sea diver clamps on his pressurized helmet before descending. Air was forced into the supposedly airtight plastic helmet, and, through "positive pressure," this air was forced into my lungs and, just as forcibly, pulled out by suction. It was uncomfortable and unpleasant in the extreme, frightening and loud. A new, and blessedly short-lived, invention of the time, the headpiece was considered a wonderful device. It made it possible to pull my body on its pallet out of the iron lung for body care.

Nursing was, in fact, extremely difficult. I could not bear to have my limbs or body touched, not even by a bedsheet, much less a washcloth. Yet, nursing training insisted upon a daily sponge bath, even at the height of the crisis. Other nursing chores were done as my body lay exposed. It was necessary to change my bladder catheter regularly, so that urine crystals did not form upon it and become the basis of infections and stones. Crystals did, however, form, and the urethra of my penis became a bloody pulp, as the catheters were inserted and withdrawn. It was, for some reason, considered important that my feet be kept upright; otherwise, dropfoot or some such thing might be expected—and this, too, caused me extreme discomfort, as my feet were wedged against a footboard. I must have been able to drink water, although I have no clear memory of this. I know that for the first two weeks or so, I did not eat, but was sustained by glucose and blood transfusions. Later, I learned that all the blood I consumed, and more, was donated by my Haverford classmates.

As the battle went on, day after day, all emotions began to fade, and a general overwhelming fatigue set in. I was literally "burnt out." I was burnt out and felt it. My state became almost serene. Things, details, lost their importance before the overwhelming big question, which was simplicity itself: stop or go, yes or no, live or die. I finally decided to live.

The decision did not come at once. It was never an affirmative decision. It was a negative one: I do not choose to die, not yet. This not-yet business was, for a while, a minute-to-minute matter, until the minutes became hours, the hours became days—until gradually, the question receded from my present consciousness.

One specific event entered into my decision. It was a rainy day. My parents were standing in the rain outside the window of my little quarantine barracks room. I remember their faces as they stood in the rain. The window had a flyscreen across it, and the rectangular lines of the screen and the gauzelike shading it gave their image remains in my memory. This screen and the rain are an inherent part of the pathetic quality.

My parents were not allowed to visit me often, perhaps not more than once or twice a day for a few minutes. I know that I had been waiting for them because I wished to say good-bye. I had had last rites. I was very tired, and I wanted them to understand that, although I was dying, I was doing so only because I could carry on the struggle no longer. I loved them very much, and I wished them to understand that I was content. My mother is a silent woman, unable to feel or express her emotions. Her love for me and my sister is, perhaps, the central focus of her life. My sister tells me that mother spent the two weeks of the crisis seated on a straight-back chair in the small lobby of the quarantine building, "awaiting developments." She did not cry; she did not talk about what was happening. She was as polite, responsive, and courteous as her son. But she would not leave. This must be kept in mind as I tell what happened next.

As I told her good-bye, a look passed over my mother's face. It was one of heartbreaking, devastating loss. Even so, she did not cry. She said something to the effect that I should hang on for another day; think about it. Perhaps things would look different, would be different tomorrow. I cannot remember what it was she said, exactly. I am certain it was said in virtually a normal conversational tone. I cannot forget, nor will I ever, the look of loss that crossed her face. And so, I replied, "All right, one more day." I groaned to myself, "Oh, Christ, one more day." I did not want one more day. As I had awaited their arrival before going to the infirmary, here I had awaited their arrival before letting go, before giving up the ghost. The thought of continuing the struggle longer, as long as another day, was difficult to bear, but I had told my mother I would do so, and I would—as I had tried to please her in every way at every time throughout my 20 years.

By this pledge to my mother, I sentenced myself to life, although I may not have been fully aware of the pledge's importance at the time. I decided to live, not because I wanted to, but because I did not want to cause my mother pain. It is a strange reason that does not bear analysis. My responsibility to myself, my essential liberty to make my own choices, was so little developed that I gave this most important decision of all to a woman standing at the window, looking through the screen, outside my room in the rain.

Certainly, giving up the ghost seemed very simple indeed. Nothing to it. Stop trying to live, and death would envelop one in warmth, comfort, and release. The struggle would be over and all would be well. I could see death clearly: it was a dark cave, warm and inviting, and I stood at its threshold. One step further, and I would be inside; I could lie down, curl up, and go to sleep. It is said that people who freeze to death experience similar sensations in the final stage—all they wish to do is lie down upon the ice, curl up, and go to sleep.

The dichotomy, which I experienced throughout my illness—one part of me experiencing the real pain, the reality; the other part somehow suspended above it all, observing—did at this point draw together, the closer I came to death. Until, standing at the threshold of the dark, warm cave, I was no longer divided between reality and observer; I was reunited as me, whole, joined in a normal manner, mind and body. It was as though my body had receded from the reality of iron lungs, pain, and crystallized catheters, had receded to join the observer, which had floated above me for these days. The two would become one, and I—free, reconstituted, whole—would step over the threshold into a new consciousness.

Although the cave was dark, there was no sense whatsoever of it's being an end to things—simply the sense of the cave entrance as a doorway. One step through the door would take me into a different consciousness. I knew instinctively at the time that the step would be irrevocable—one step over, no step back possible, ever. This knowledge was what produced the strong desire to say good-bye to my parents. I might say it was like taking a trip, waving good-bye as the ship pulls away from the dock. But it was not, for people return from voyages. Even if they do not, they live on the same planet, and they write letters to each other. They are still there, reachable.

Death was different. It was not like the voyage. It was final. It was similar, although quite different, to the effect of hallucinogenic drugs. It was a very definite entering of another state of consciousness. On a drug trip, however, there is—or has always been for me—the sense that what goes up will come down, that what is being experienced will not last. Whatever is going on inside the head, one knows the outside world remains, and the body and mind remain firmly based within it. In death, mind and body seemed to go together. There was nothing artificial, temporary, or induced. It just was there, natural, inevitable, all right. It was the next step.

This experience has, of course, lived with me for 25 years. I think about it often. It has altered significantly my attitude toward life and toward death—both mine and that of my family and friends. I was extremely neurotic, ambitious, a super-achiever, if ever there was one. And I still am. However, since my experience with death in the iron lung in Bryn Mawr Hospital, the things of this earth—and I love things dearly—the things of this earth do not have the importance for me, which I see others attaching to them. There is a perspective about living and dying. I think those who have experienced it are made different by the experience. It is a difference that can be felt more easily than expressed; it is an experience that can be forgotten in the hurley-burley, the hassle, of the day's events, in the rush of one's ambition and work. It can be forgotten, but it can never be lost; and, in times of crisis when exams and promotions and deadlines take over the importance of life, the experience will reassert itself. The experience is a lesson; there is a simplicity to life, a beauty to death, and the fact of living is too important, short, and fragile to be shoved aside by self-inflicted fissions and failures.

And so, all unknowing, I lived.

In the Franz Kafka's *Metamorphosis*, the man wakes up to find himself encased in the body of a cockroach. And so, after two weeks of drama, I woke up to find myself imprisoned in an iron lung. After two weeks, my temperature receded, returned to normal. The blood transfusions, the glucose feedings were halted. The vigil at the doors of death was called off, and ordinary hospital life began.

I, my lung and I, was moved out of the quarantine building into a private room. My six nurses went with me and remained with me for close to three months. The lung was positioned in the room so that, reflected in my mirror, I could see people walking down the hospital corridor when the door to my room was open. I do not know whether there was a view from my window, for, in the three months I was to occupy the room, I never once was in a position to look out the window. A television set, not then standard equipment for hospital rooms, was bought or rented. One of my nurses was a great fan of Robin Roberts, a pitcher then with the Philadelphia Phillies. It was summer; the room was not air conditioned. In my memory, it seems the television was always on, the channel always tuned to baseball. Seen through my mirror, the game was, of course, reversed. A home run would send the runner from home to third, to second, to first, and back again to home plate. I have never cared much for baseball, nor did I care for it then; however, the sameness of it, the constancy of play, the familiarity of the summer baseball crowd sounds were soothing and oddly comforting.

My skin was still exceedingly sensitive; my limbs were still frozen with muscular adhesions; my body was still paralyzed from head to foot. Eyesight, swallowing, sense of smell had returned to normal. I was no longer breathing pure oxygen through my tracheotomy tube.

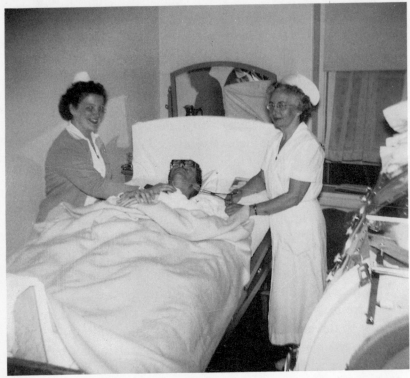

This was taken the first day my lungs were strong enough to allow me to be moved from the iron lung to a hospital bed. Evil nurse McGranahan stands between me and the lung. I am lying flat because muscular adhesions are so tight, I cannot be bent without great pain. Note I am wearing eye glasses made of prisms which allow me to see around the room without moving or lifting my head.

The oxygen tank was kept on standby in case of emergencies, but I was once again breathing air, still, though, through the tracheotomy.

Nursing care within the lung was exceedingly difficult for the nurses and painful to me. The lung was built like a submarine, neatly riveted with round portholes along the side, a sausage-shaped window above the portholes. There was along the side a hatch, which could be opened for the insertion of such necessities as bedpan, soap, and water. These would be placed inside and the hatch resealed. The nurses would insert their arms through the opened portholes, do whatever needed doing to my body, watching the operation through the sausage-shaped window. The portholes were lined with a rubber cuff, and, in theory, the nurses' arms, tightly cuffed, would not break the vacuum and weaken the pressure achieved by the pump. Like many a theory, the practice was considerably less effective than the concept. There was always difficulty maintaining the pressure within the lung; the collar around my neck constantly chafed, always leaked. Wads of cotton were stuffed into the gaps. These would withstand the pressure for a bit, but then, on the intake stroke, be sucked—small white projectiles—imploding to the foot of the respirator. These drops in pressure would result in shallow breaths, half-filled lungs. It was annoying, frightening, to be robbed of expected air through circumstances outside one's body.

For weeks, the nurses and I had to struggle with Sister Kenny's hot packs. Sister Kenny, an Australian nurse, revolutionized the post-crisis treatment of polio. Before her time, doctors had insisted that patients be left immobile, sometimes even encasing them in plaster. This not only resulted in obvious foreseeable atrophy of whatever motor power was left to the surviving muscles, but also ensured that muscle adhesions turned from stiffness to concrete. Sister Kenny insisted upon a regime designed to keep the muscles as loose, relaxed, and flexible as possible. She called for physical therapy range-of-motion exercises for the limbs as soon as the critical period was over. Part of her program was hot packs.

Hot packs were old surplus Army blankets, cut into squares, dunked in boiling water, and wrapped around the limbs. They were supposed to soothe and comfort the aching muscles, reduce the inflammation, and, no doubt, other good things. They were, in fact, if not a torture, certainly a major nuisance.

A summer's day in Philadelphia, a hospital room crowded with equipment, an iron lung, and an oxygen tank. To this, add a clothes-line, a hot plate, and buckets of boiling water. The blanket squares were dropped into the water, fished out with calipers, hung to cool a bit, inserted through the hatch, and draped appropriately about my body. I was too stiff, too immobile, in too much pain, actually, to have my limbs wrapped; they were simply draped. The process, repeated throughout the day, made a hot room very hot and the harried nurses' day even more harassed.

The packs were the work of my physical therapist. She was the only true sadist I have ever known. There can be no excuse whatsoever for the terror and fear she caused me. It was her charge over the ensuing weeks to wean me from the respirator, as the muscles used for breathing regained their strength. It was her responsibility to see that the adhesions in my joints were broken up, my tight muscles stretched to a full range of flexibility. These are painful processes; in no way can they be considered easy. Even with the closest cooperation between patient and therapist, even with the greatest patient confidence in his therapist, the process will be arduous, painful. Granted this, there can be no excuse for the cruel, vicious, and inhumane manner with which my therapist proceeded with her tasks. She did nothing whatsoever to introduce me to pain and how to handle it; she did nothing to gain my trust; she early lost my confidence.

To my real pain and legitimate apprehension, she added a whole new level of sadistic torture, a torture that I am certain gave her a significant degree of pleasure. This woman is now dead. I can only hope that she is roasting in hell, roommates with that Nazi woman who made lampshades out of the skins of her concentration camp victims.

With the exception of an older cranky nurse, who was to become mixed up in my bowel problems, my nurses were a cheerful, pleasant, dedicated crew. Every one of them during the crisis worked very, very, hard. All of them had a real and personal commitment to my recovery. They nursed me with a deep concern, which I am certain drained them emotionally, as well as physically. I will always be grateful to them. Particularly grateful am I to a young girl, who nursed me on the night shift—buxom and cheerful, dark-haired and bright-eyed, she would lean over me, her bosom pressed against my head, in the wee hours of the night. We would exchange stories of our hopes and plans: she to marry her boyfriend, then at war in Korea; me—what for me? What dreams did I tell her? I told her about the mountains, about Colorado, about a girl I had loved, about the kind of life I would lead. I told her these things; there were other things I did not tell her.

Once I had moved out of quarantine, my mother returned to my life. She had spent the crisis weeks sitting in the anteroom of the quarantine building. Now, she was allowed into my room, where she would sit on a chair beside the respirator. My father and sister returned to Washington to job and school. They would come to Philadelphia on weekends to spell and assist my mother. My mother remained with me. She would arrive in the morning after breakfast and stay throughout the day, leaving only with one of my special duty nurses, Miss McGranahan, when she went off shift at 11 in the evening. Mother was boarding with the McGranahans.

Mother never talked about what was happening to my body. She never shared with me the emotional distress she had felt during the crisis, nor did she ever let me know that she was aware of the stress, the catastrophic stress through which I was moving. Mother was never able to express emotions. Indeed, I have not the least idea what she felt, ever. She simply was there, always cheerful, constant, sociable—always these, but never more than these. She was simply there. Poor woman, I had literary pretensions in those days. From beside the respirator, she would read to me. I remember she read an article by the Texas author, J. Frank Dobie, from the current *Atlantic Monthly*. I was particularly interested in the article, whatever it was about; mother would read it to me. She had to read it over and over because I would drift off to sleep before it was well begun and awake only when her voice would cease. Like a ritualized lullaby, I slept as mother read, as mother read aloud the *Atlantic Monthly*.

There were many visitors from the college—my classmates, my professors. In particular, my ethics instructor, Dr. Martin Foss, came to me on a regular basis. He was a good and gentle man of profound sensitivity. He and his wife had come to this country as refugees. They had been interned in a Nazi concentration camp, an experience from which his wife had never fully regained her sanity. Of all my visitors, he alone had the empathy and awareness to share with me my hurt, my loss. He was magnificent.

With the advent of summer, the college semester came to a close, and my classmates went off upon their way. One of them came to say good-bye, bringing me a vast bouquet of flowers. "Oh," I said, "you should not have." He smiled, "Actually, I haven't," he said sheepishly. "These are from my grandmother's funeral." I told the story to other visitors, and they found it amusing. It was one of a variety of anecdotes I had found with which to entertain my visitors. I myself did not find it funny at all.

There was such a vast invasion of privacy—a destruction of all privacy. One day my lover came to say good-bye, and there is my mother and there are the nurses. There is the iron lung, the body that will not move, the lungs that will not work. I cannot write. I cannot sneak off for a phone call. I cannot hold a phone to my ear. I cannot talk at all, unless someone places a finger over the tracheotomy pipe. I cannot pee; I cannot shit. I cannot masturbate; I cannot stroke or see myself. All my life, I have been a person who can only handle my emotions in privacy; now, I am a person without privacy. A child who achieved separation from his parents only after the greatest effort, I now find myself thrust back, dependent upon my mother, dependent upon my father. Throughout the whole experience, there is no privacy, nor is there anyone with whom to share the emotional impact of my experience. As cheerful of demeanor as my mother, I continue pleasant and helpful, certainly the most popular patient on the floor. It is a wonder I did not turn catatonic with suppressed rage and grief.

I was raped at some point during the week. I was forcibly violated in a particularly horrible and humiliating manner. My nurse, Miss McGranahan, was a stern lady, who brooked no foolishness and was most concerned with bowels and constipation. During the period of crisis, I had been too sick for normal nursing. As a result, I developed bedsores, the scars of which I carry to this day. I also developed a fecal impaction of the bowels. I was at first too weak to shit, and soon the shit was so firmly packed that my feeble bowels could not evacuate themselves, even with the stimulation of severe cathartics, even with the insistent encouragement of enemas. There are, I understand, means by which this condition may be remedied. They are, I believe, unpleasant, but effective. They were not used on me.

One evening, Miss McGranahan put on her rubber gloves, turned me on my side, pried open my rectum, reached in and ripped out the fecal matter, piece by piece. She did it without warning and without explanation; she did it without sedatives or anesthesia. She left me powerless, impotent, reduced to tears of despair. She was herself renewed in triumph and power. I hated her. Furthermore, I hated her with a hate I could express to no one, for I was too humiliated to tell my story. The emotions she had aroused were too awful for a person raised as I had been, to feel, let alone express, to others or even to myself. By this one act, Miss McGranahan set up problems with sexuality and problems with authority, which I have yet to resolve satisfactorily.

Until then, I do not believe I had ever thought much about bowel movements. They had been more or less natural, regular occurrences, providing little pleasure, no pain, just a part of living. Now they had become, and would remain, a nightmare. Even with laxatives and enemas, my bowels worked poorly. Calling for a bedpan was more than embarrassing; so thin and sensitive was I that it was a painful experience. Even with sponge rubber taped to the pan's metal rim, even with pillows surrounding, it was a hurtful business, and I dreaded it.

Over time and very slowly, some of my muscles began to regain strength and movement. My right hand, now shaky and weak, was able to function, although it was many months before the thumb on my right hand was able to resume its critical opposing position. With the knuckle of my right hand, now I could knock on the side of the iron lung when I wished to speak. This was a signal to my nurses to place an index finger over the tracheotomy hole, so that I could make use of my vocal cords.

As the weeks went by, it became crucial that I begin to show signs of a return of my breathing response. In order, so she said, to test for this, my therapist took to dropping in on me in the night hours, unaware. Returning from a dinner party, she would stop by, hoping to catch me asleep. Finding me asleep, she would turn off the respirator and, with a stopwatch, time how long it was before I awoke from suffocation. At this point, laughing, she would turn the respirator back on and proceed upon her way. The sense of waking to suffocation as a result of these games is another thing I carry with me to this day. I do not like to be awakened quickly, unexpectedly at night, by telephone or doorbell—as, for an instant, in the dark, I am once again in the respirator, suffocating to death, crying out for help, with no one to hear because my vocal cords without air cannot sound. When I am awakened suddenly at night, for a second I am trapped, paralyzed, mute, and dying. It is an awful feeling.

The hospital routine was not unpleasant. The room was bright and cheerful. My nurses were pleasant, my mother ever-present. Although my father was at the hospital only on weekends, he displayed an emotional concern, which I find a good thing to recall. The day was filled with things to be done. The miserable hot packs had to be put on and taken off. My lungs had to be aspirated through the silver tube of my tracheotomy several times a day; my bowels had to be attended to; a daily sponge bath involved complicated maneuvering to get pans and soap inside the respirator while maintaining adequate air pressure. During this period, I was eating and drinking fluids, but I have no memory as to their quality or kinds. There were regular visitors. Particularly do I remember the Episcopal priest, who had given me last rites, called regularly to administer communion; and, of course, Martin Foss was faithful in his attendance.

There was a rhythm to the day, a rhythm set by the throbbing pump of the respirator, ever present like the throb of the steamer's engines as it churns across the sea. To the beat of the iron lung was imposed the artificial division of the day into thirds, each third presaged by the arrival of a new shift of nurses. In memory, it seems to be always evening, twilight, with the lights going on up and down the corridor, the murmur and moans of other patients and visitors—the busy, subdued, but living sounds of a hospital. My world had collapsed—it had spread from Europe to California, from the constraints of my mother's living room to the unlimited dimensions of my new-found life at Haverford. It had been that big, and it was now confined to an iron lung in a hospital room. This did not mean it was less interesting, less adventuresome, less challenging—for surely it was interesting, adventuresome, and challenging in the extreme. It was just that little things expanded in importance. Things that had been automatic and unconsciously done—breathing, bowels, bladder—now took on major importance, had become difficult and challenging.

There is a Parkinsonian aspect to life in an iron lung—things compact, as well as expand, and whatever is available will fill the time and attention.

Breathing took much of my attention. At first, I had to learn how to breathe *with* the respirator. This experience can be frightening; inhale when the machine says exhale, and the result is confusion, mixed with an impotent fear. Once one learns to breathe with the machine, being in an iron lung becomes oddly comforting. It is warm, life-sustaining; its steel body protects you from the dangers of living, of breathing. It is a big womb, an overprotective mommy, and, as I was led to believe, can become as deadly habit-forming an addiction as any drug.

I learned one evening just how dangerous and deadly it could be. Mother was down the hall in the waiting room, and my two nurses were getting me ready for sleep. I had been in the respirator three weeks; everyone had decided that I was going to live after all, but no one knew how much longer I would need the iron lung. I could breathe for only a few seconds without becoming panicky, and I was still getting air through the half-inch tracheotomy tube in my throat. I was no longer breathing pure oxygen, had not done so for three days, but the tank was still kept in the corner of the room, just in case. My FM radio was playing, I remember, Brahms' Third Symphony.

The slow, rhythmic whoosh of the respirator had become a part of my world; it was in the background, ever present, day and night. The whoosh was keeping me alive in the iron and steel, warm and protective womb of the respirator. I had complete confidence in it.

My nurses, Miss McGranahan and Miss Johnson, were assembling the back-rubbing equipment in preparation for what was the painful task of turning me on my side for a back rub. And then the respirator stopped. It stopped with the crispness of snow on a still, cold night.

It stopped with a thundering quiet that bounced from the blank hospital walls. With my last full breath, I whispered, "It's stopped," and the rasp came from my stomach and out the tube, leaving my lips empty and moving.

My nurses leapt into action, looking as though they were not quite sure where to leap. Miss McGranahan shouted, "Keep calm, Hugh, keep calm!" and rushed to the rear of the lung where there was a manual pump. She heaved and pushed frantically at the pump handle, moving it a few inches in and a few inches out, but, as there was not time for her to read the instruction plate in front of her nose, she never saw the lever that had to be turned to free the handle for manual operation. She heaved, she pushed, with all the strength a 56-year old spinster who repairs her own car, can achieve. That the handle, bellows and all, did not come off in her hand is, indeed, a tribute to the manufacturer. I am sure Miss

McGranahan had never worked so hard nor so ineffectively. The air pressure of the lung never varied.

"Keep calm, keep calm," she shrieked. I was breathing in short little gasps, using the muscles of my neck to expand my chest. I could not have lasted more than five minutes. Breathing took my every effort. I had no time to do anything but keep calm.

Miss Johnson, in the meantime, was on the phone. She started with a high-pitched, "HELP!," that slid down into a shouted nonstop, "Electricianelectricianelectrician!" Slamming down the receiver, she made for the oxygen tank. I remember thinking, at last, here comes some real help. The tank was almost as tall as Miss Johnson and was built in roughly the same shape. The two wrestled each other across the floor to the lung. Miss Johnson put the oxygen hose in my tracheotomy tube.

"Keep calm!" Miss McGranahan shrieked, "Calm everybody!" as she pumped mightily at the pump that pumped nothing. The tube was in place, but there was no oxygen. Miss Johnson maintains to this day that the tank was out of gas; I suspect she forgot to open the valve.

At any rate, at that moment, the door was flung open. Standing in the doorway was the head nurse, who possessed as much dignity as the late Dowager Queen Mary and was certainly far more severe. Obviously in a great temper, she stood there and said firmly, slowly, and with finality, "Turn down that radio."

"Calm!" Miss McGranahan screeched. "Help!" shouted Miss Johnson. The head nurse had never been shouted at before in her life, I'm sure. "Can't you see it's stopped? Go get help; don't just stand there." As an afterthought, my nurse added, "Keep calm!" I doubt that the head nurse heard it, for as soon as she saw what had happened, she trotted off for help.

The respirator started again roughly four minutes after it had stopped. It began as it had ceased without warning or reason. The electrician arrived, wearing an overcoat over his pajamas. He checked over the lung wiring for a long time and could find nothing wrong. The head nurse arrived with two interns and a resident who checked me over for a long time and could find nothing wrong. Miss McGranahan had to sit down. She looked perilously close to hysteria.

On the way to the elevator, the electrician tells me, he met my mother. She started when she saw him, saying, "Anything wrong, is there anything wrong?"

"No," he said, "just checking," and went back home to bed.

I was, once established on the iron lung routine, reasonably comfortable and not anxious to alter my circumstances. This was a feeling not shared by others. My doctors, my therapist, and my nurses were extremely anxious that I be weaned from the respirator. After the onset of polio, it is weeks, months, before a pattern of muscle recovery can be established. At the beginning, no one can tell whether the nerves that direct the muscles have been killed or simply injured. So it was that no one could tell whether I would recover the ability to breathe free of the machine. The life expectancy of patients in iron lungs was not good. A simple cold was a crisis; pneumonia was fatal. A recovered polio, with reasonable lung power, had a future—not without obstacles, but he had a future.

As the days in the respirator turned into weeks, the anxieties felt by all began to build. My Prussian therapist put me on a breathing schedule which, when imposed, seemed, quite simply, impossible. She wished me to breathe for 30 seconds without the assistance of the respirator. At first, this meant, once the lung was turned off, that I would go for 30 seconds without taking a real breath, without new oxygen being introduced into the lungs. It was not that I did not try; it was simply that the muscles were not responding to my directions. I did, in heavy concentration, direct myself to breathe; my directions simply elicited no response from my diaphragm or intercostal muscles.

After several days, I cannot be sure how long, perhaps a week or two, she began to up the stakes. I had learned to take a breath, perhaps two. Now, she said, the time would be doubled from 30 seconds to a minute. After I had breathed a minute, the time would be upped to two minutes; and then she said, each day's time would be doubled. Two minutes today, four minutes tomorrow, eight minutes the next, sixteen minutes the following, and so on. After I was able to breathe 10 minutes on my own, the pallet on which I was lying would be pulled out from my respirator, and my nurses would be able to attend to my body needs directly instead of poking their arms through the inadequate portholes. After I was able to breathe an hour without assistance, I would be lifted and placed, for that time period, upon a bed free from the respirator. She said, and it seemed wildly, wildly impossible, that by the time I was able to breathe for three hours without help, I would not want to return to the lung. Last, she said that once I learned to sleep a whole night through outside the lung, I would never need or wish to return to it.

As this was told to me, it seemed impossible. It was like telling a goldfish it could walk. Each day through my little mirror, I could see people passing the door of my room, breathing, talking, laughing. They seemed to do these things with a natural ease that astonished me. While it is true that for 20 years, I, too, had done these things, now I had forgotten how. Of course, I was paralyzed, but I had also forgotten *how* to go about breathing without conscious effort or strain. As an astronaut upon the moon is dependent upon his space suit, so was I dependent upon my iron lung. I would fight any effort to separate me from my lung with all the perseverance with which I had hung on to life. I envied the breathers, but I did not think that I would ever be one of them again.

So it was that I started—started on the long, unending effort to recover and maintain my body strengths. The therapist's plan went like clockwork. The driving schedule, just one more painful and frightening event in the day, went on inexorably. Somehow, the muscles that were responsible for breathing were able to meet the challenge. I was actually breathing on my own—first, for no more than a few minutes a day, then by leaps and bounds, for longer periods. We were able to do away with the horrible crashing diver's helmet, which hitherto had clamped over my head whenever nursing required cutting off the pressure. Some five weeks after I was placed in the respirator, I was, for the first time, moved out of it onto a bed alongside.

This was, for me, a day of very great achievement. No personal accomplishment has given me greater pride. There was satisfaction, mixed with increasing hope through evidence, that recovery was possible; indeed, recovery was occurring. It was heady intoxication. I was on the bed for less than an hour. It took four or five people to effect the transfer. My body was still rigid with muscular adhesions; the least deflection of my limbs from the horizontal produced intense, exquisite pain. I had not been aware, until I was moved, just how painful and sensitive my body still was. The move was an agony I had not expected, nor did I expect the extreme fatigue that overcame me, once I had been breathing on my own, totally away from the lung for an hour. The sheer exertion of breathing was such that, upon being returned to the respirator, I slept for the rest of the afternoon, relieved to be back in the warmth and comfort of my familiar prison. It takes a while for the prisoner to adjust to freedom.

Now that I was out of the respirator—and soon enough I was out of it altogether—sleeping outside the lung proved to be less difficult than I had expected. So much effort was expended in breathing that it was easy enough to drift off into restful sleep unaided. Now that I was out on a bed, my therapist had room to begin full range of motion exercises with my limbs. These are simple. The limb is lifted and moved through the pattern of normal extension. Because, however, of the extreme tightness around my muscles, even such simple exercises were painful. Since those early days, I have learned how to live with pain, how to go with it, how to accept it, rather than fight. Fighting pain, anticipating it, fearing it, simply makes it worse. Resistance and anxiety make pain more painful. This is not a lesson I learned from my therapist. She did, in fact, everything possible to heighten my fear and increase my pain. It was her job to stretch out my limbs and to bring flexibility back to my body. I understood that. She did her job in a sadistic way. When she was stretching my hamstrings, she would say, "Tell me when the pain is as much as you can take, and then we will count to 10, and then I will release my pressure." She would take me through to the threshold of extreme pain. I would tell her; she would count to 10, but, then, she would not release the pressure—she would push harder for another five seconds or so. She took a devilish sort of glee in this sneaky attempt to inflict just a little more stretching, just a little more pain. She had another trick. When she was talking to me or to a third party in the room, without warning, her arm would dart out, and she would grab my wrist, yanking my stiff and painful arm into the air and giving it a brutal jerk. This sort of thing really does very little to loosen up tight muscles. It only serves to increase the patient's anxiety and pain.

My father, impressed by the therapist's strong will, had allied himself with her. He mistakenly believed that such tactics were part of what was required for my convalescence. I know now they were not.

At the time, I had been so demoralized by my condition, so brain-washed by doctors, nurses, and this Prussian therapist, that I had lost all sense of property rights over my own body. It seemed to belong to them; they knew best, I was always being told. It was my duty to accept what they said and do what they said to do, for they were all working in my best interests.

And, so, I was trying my best, and the pains and hurts, which I had hoped would be receding, did not recede. My bowels were still causing me pain and anxiety; my lungs still needed constant aspiration. The catheter, which passed through the urethra of my penis, had to be changed frequently; my urethra was sliced to bloody ribbons. Crystals, which had formed upon the catheter, developed into kidney and bladder stones, and my urinary tract was infected. Stretching and therapy were agony, and the anxiety of my constant vigilance against unexpected pain was exhausting. One afternoon, I could take it no longer.

My father and therapist were at the bed. My chief doctor, a neurologist/psychiatrist named Bartel, came in. The two retreated. I was in exhausted pain, and I needed encouragement. For weeks, now over two months, I had taken what was handed to me without complaint. I did so, believing that full cooperation was the price of getting well. The pain and the torture inflicted upon me by nurses, doctors, and therapists attending to my various conditions were part of the treatment. The treatment was the means, the vehicle, by which I would move from sickness to health. There would be an end to it, I felt; and, somehow, I had formed the belief that it would be over by the end of summer, that I would be able to return to school in the fall. In the fall, I felt I would get back to being *me*.

It had not occurred to me that I might not "get well"; it had not yet occurred to me that I might have residual paralysis, that I might remain crippled. After all, I had no experience with permanent injury. Always before when I had been sick, I had, after a suitable period, become well. I was a person of inordinate vanity; I disliked cripples—they were to me as lepers. They were unclean, broken. I looked upon them with revulsion. They had nothing to do with my life. Through my teenage years, I had constructed my body as carefully as I did my studies or chose my wardrobe—very carefully. That this polio should not end was unthinkable. That this polio should leave me with permanent paralysis was unacceptable. Oh, I was game. I could take all the pain and treatment the doctors could hand out. But there would be an end point; there must be a goal. I would return to Haverford in the fall, fully restored in body and health. I would be fully restored, too, in the independence of mind and control over my own body, which I had lost during the illness.

And, so, Dr. Bartel came upon me one afternoon in the middle of my physical therapy session. In my exasperation, seeking encouragement, I asked him some questions about my condition; and I asked these questions point blank. For the first time, he answered them. He was both direct and kindly. I see now that he was as positive and optimistic as the circumstances permitted. All that I remember that he specifically said was that I would never again walk without assistance. He spoke of the possibility of crutches, braces, Canadian canes, perhaps in time, no more than a cane or so.

It may be that these things were said to me before. It may be they were said to me often. I know only on that afternoon, I acknowledged to myself for the first time that everything had changed. I would never again be beautiful, innocent, secure in health, strong in body, confident in mind. Everything had changed, and I would be forever crippled. Bartel left the room; the therapist and my father returned—the exercises, the stretching, the hurt were begun anew.

I had hysterics. Never before nor since have I been hysterical in quite that way. Like other frightening things, it is much worse in expectation than it is in fact. Its approach is the dreadful business: the bottling up of impossible passions and emotions, the struggling to contain the feelings that are exploding with you—that is the dreadful part. The hysterics, the release, once triggered, is unstoppable; but with the triggering, there comes the sense that the self will not, indeed cannot, take any more. A line is drawn, and this is it. Nothing more can be received or handled by the emotions. The body protects itself, and there is a limit to sanity. This limit had at long last been reached.

A look came upon my father's face, which I do not forget. During my illness, he had busied himself, consulting doctors from coast to coast, being efficient and businesslike, seeing to it that everything that could be done was done. He had traveled back and forth from Washington under strenuous, self-imposed circumstances. He had accepted the value structure of the physical therapist and had joined her in the tortures, which he had been told were necessary. I think, in those moments of my hysteria, he realized for the first time—I think he felt for the first time and, perhaps, for the only time he allowed himself to feel—the full extent of my hurt. His face was transparent to the emotions behind it; he saw the ghastly impotence of my condition. It was as though his eyes had looked into hell itself. And he left me; he left the room.

The effect of my behavior upon everyone was immediate and electric. Nurses and doctors and earnest young interns ran about. They did not allow it to run its course; they did not allow me to let it all come out as a good and sensible reaction to the monstrous, nonsensible things that had happened to me. They treated my hysterics as something shameful, embarrassing, something to be hidden, to be throttled as quickly as possible. I was given a shot of something, which produced an almost immediate and beatific calming result. Orders were given, remonstrances heard, and people stopped hurting me.

For at least 48 hours, I had a surcease from the pain imposed upon me by the medical, nursing, and therapy regimes. And, afterwards, as it was necessary to pick up again the treatment, it was picked up with a certain respect for my feelings and an acknowledgment of my person. Never again have I let myself be treated as solely "patient material." Never again have I allowed myself and my integrity to be invaded and raped by outsiders. My hysteria was an eminently suitable, rational response to a dreadful situation. Although the hysteria itself was wildly beyond rationality, the final collapse of the rational controls, which had allowed me to retain for so long the horrors of my situation, did produce the results required. The cost, however, was very high.

My father had seen and, perhaps, momentarily shared my despair and suffering. He was repulsed by it, repelled by it. And he retreated from the room. He did not reach out his hand, he did not hold me, he did not weep with me—he left me alone. I learned again that day that an expression of my honest emotions and feelings was not acceptable. There was something disgusting about them and, thus, about me. My honest feelings must be hidden from my family, those who loved me. If I showed even a fraction of the depth of my feelings, they would abandon me; they would leave the room. This experience had been repeated time and again in my childhood until I had learned to hide everything behind the slipcovers of polite convention. Now, finally, in emotional extremism, I had ripped through the slipcovers, reaching out in my desperate need. They had responded in horror and had left the room. I was ashamed and abandoned.

The young man I had been, rich in life and youth, died that afternoon. Hope and love died that afternoon. I retreated into myself, much as the "good" Germans went into "internal exile" through the Nazi years. I became again the cheerful patient, the dutiful son. I cooperated with the doctors, the nurses, the therapists. And the hurts and pains continued and, gradually, they lessened. The muscles in my hands and arms and shoulders gradually returned—very, very gradually. There was definite improvement in my condition when measured week by week, month by month. But, so far as I was concerned, so far as the real me was concerned, it did not matter—none of it mattered. It was all over. I had retreated into a private place, deep within me.

They could hurt my body; they could insult my person; they could abandon me; they could deny the integrity of my feelings and refuse to acknowledge my legitimate emotions, but they could not hurt me, for I was not there. That afternoon, when I had hysterics, I said, never again. I might have looked and sounded like the same person, but I was not. I would not, I could not take such hurt and rejection again. I would not allow myself to feel it. This required me to stop feeling altogether, for as I was unwilling to feel the shame and despair, just so I must give up all feelings—deny them all. I became that day a physical, emotional clone. Polio had its victory that day for I gave up. From then on, they could do anything they liked to me. I would do anything they asked, but I had fooled them. I would not be there. I had gone far, far away. There was no way they could reach me, no way they could touch me, not one of them, ever, even if one should really try.

The summer passed, and it was time to go home. I was not well enough, of course, to leave the hospital, but I was considered well enough to make the journey to Washington. A hospital, doctors, and nurses were located in Washington; travel arrangements of great complexity were worked out. Three months after I had entered, I left Bryn Mawr Hospital. I had come on a stretcher, and I left on a stretcher. The crisis was over. The disease had receded; I could breathe on my own again. I could swallow; I could see; I had some use of my right hand and the fingers on my left hand. I would live.

However, my condition was still grave. I had virtually no cough reflex. I still had the silver tracheotomy tube in my throat, and I still required constant aspiration to clear my lungs of fluid. I had developed a stone in my right kidney, and I had a large stone and gravel in my bladder. A urinary infection was quiescent but not gone. I was not yet strong enough to withstand surgery; and, as the stones were too large to pass of their own accord, they were left where they were. Stones are painful enough, but they are not fatal, not immediately.

My body was still extremely sensitive; the muscle adhesions had just begun to be broken up, and I was stiff as a board. I could not bear bending, no matter how slight. I was extremely weak. The least amount of movement, excitement, or worry caused me great tortures of anxiety. Polio, of course, is a disease of the central nervous system. Not only were my nerves sensitive, but also that portion of the nervous system related to the emotions was gravely harmed and only recovering slowly. Because of the possibility of some crisis unforeseen—physical or emotional—it was decided by my doctors that I could not travel without a respirator, oxygen tanks, aspirating equipment, and medical attendants. All of this required the rental of a private railroad car.

The car was pulled up at a siding when I arrived in the ambulance. Very gently, my stretcher was lifted onto the platform, and I watched with fascination as workmen in railroad overalls unscrewed a window of the Pullman car. Because of the narrow corridor at the ends of the car, it was necessary to remove a window so that my stretcher could be lifted directly into the car. This was done; the window was replaced; my mother and the nurses entered the Pullman. My car was attached to the tail-end of a New York-to-Washington bound train.

At Union Station, I was met by my father, my sister, and my dog, Tigger. I had not seen Tigger since I had entered the hospital. There were two reporters and a photographer present. I answered their questions in a cheerful, confident manner. The flashbulb went off; pictures were taken.

My stretcher was wheeled through the vast concourse of the station out through the great doors. I saw in front of me the dome of the Capitol Building, brilliant white against the blue sky of Washington. I was lifted again into an ambulance and taken off to Providence Hospital. There would be six surgical operations and more than 20 additional months of care before I was released from the hospital. And then, I was released to my parents' care, helpless as an infant boy.

I had left home to go out into the world. I had gone in search of freedom, self-worth, a growth and development of my own values, according to the passions and the emotions that were so strongly felt. I returned home, against my will, dependent, with my values, desires, and emotions locked away.

There are pictures of concentration camp victims who did not die. They have been rescued for reasons inexplicable to them—they have been rescued, and they will not die. They walk about and they talk, and they are reunited with their families. They will resume their lives, their businesses, their habits. They look at the camera in these pictures of the supreme moment of their rescue. They look unblinking, expressionless, and blank. They stare at the camera, and *there is no life to them.*

My Hospital Journal

A year ago, I came across the journal I had kept while I was at Providence Hospital, Washington, D.C., in the spring of 1953. I had completely forgotten about it. Reading it now, I feel as though I were reading someone else's diary. The neat script, so carefully written, is most unlike my writing of today. Reading on, however, I recognize the person I was, more than 40 years ago. Although much has changed, I am still that 20-year-old boy, writing his journal in his hospital bed in the old Providence Hospital.

I stayed at Providence for nine months, during which time I had seven surgical procedures for kidney stones, bladder stones, and a breast tumor. I began physical therapy. For all these months, I made do with one private nurse a shift. The bills were paid by the Polio Foundation. There was no way that my parents could have paid, short of mortgaging everything they owned. The close, attentive care I received was no luxury; I would have died without it. What would have happened to me today, what with the extraordinary rise in health care costs and the allocation of that care by health maintenance organizations, I cannot say. Certainly I would not have received the atten-

tive care I had then. My doctors and nurses worked very hard for very long keeping me alive.

Only slowly did I emerge from the land of the sick. By the spring of 1953, I had regained my ability to breathe, to swallow, to see. Muscle power was returning to my hands, arms, and shoulders. I was able to read books again without assistance, and I was able to write again with a rubber band wrapped around my hand to compensate for muscle weakness. Without it, I could not grasp my pen.

I began a journal. Reading it again, I find an innocence and a bravery that cuts me to the core. It brings back memories of my close-to-fatal determination not to think about the terrible situation in which I found myself. I had been reading Virginia Woolf's diaries. I wanted to write as honestly as Woolf, but I was not prepared to face my emotions. That would only come much later.

I was a 20-year-old boy who always tried to play by the rules. According to the male code of the day, a man kept his pain and anxiety to himself. He had self-control and self-confidence; he was always positive, and he never complained. I am no John Wayne, but I did my best to live up to his standards. Therefore, there is little complaining in my journal. Only obliquely can the reader sense the pain, physical and emotional, the fear and doubt. My diary reminds me that I really was hanging on to life and sanity by a very thin thread.

I think you will see what I mean in the following selections from my journal. The editor at Vandamere Press would like me to say they have not been edited. They are printed as I wrote them in 1953.

JANUARY 14, MONDAY

Back in Providence. And alone for first time since Friday. I didn't start this til today—I was too embarrassed and afraid that the family might tease me about it. They wouldn't, of course, but it seems so presumptive and "corny" to be writing a journal. All goes back to my tubby days when I was afraid of being laughed at.

Many times I've wished I could be as enthusiastic and water-proofed as Bill Smith. He goes off the deep end with everything he starts and he doesn't seem to care—overly—about the opinions of others. I am enthusiastic over ideas, too, but I tend to keep them hidden, away from my surface emotions.

There seems to be a contradiction here in my goals—I want always to be calm (I've worked for that for years) and on the other hand I would like to be able to become interested and excited about projects. Of course there is no real contradiction now that I look at it. My sought after serenity is no more than a mask of surface calmness covering an inner turbidness (that is a word?), a false front. What I am after is a genuine, real serenity of will and spirit. An ability to accept any happening or adversity with a calmness and a "peace of mind." I'm living thru a pretty severe test of this now, but no worse a one than many others have lived thru and mastered. This peace of mind I must not confuse with a fear of public opinion. That's pride. The trick is to be calm in the face of derision. And not to let your actions, your interests, your enthusiasms be governed by a fear of public derision. Act as you know you should and as you feel you must, keeping calm in the face of the outcome.

I am reading Thomas Merton's *Journal* in a Trappist monastery, which is the reason—the present one at least—of my starting mine. I have been wanting to keep one for years, ever since reading Somerset Maugham's and Scott Fitzgerald's, but that old fear of "what will everyone think of my presumption" sorta kept me from it. Pretty childish. (The journal might be pretty childish too!)

[Portion of journal omitted.]

I write this with a rubber band holding my thumb in place. I hope that this writing will act as a sort of therapy. Hope so as my thumb muscle is shot.

LATER.

I live in such a noisy world of man made noise. All day long, people yelling at me from the radio, screaming commercials, Sound Off for Chesterfields, Screeching on television. At times I feel as though I can't take another minute of it. And yet I am uncomfortable in the

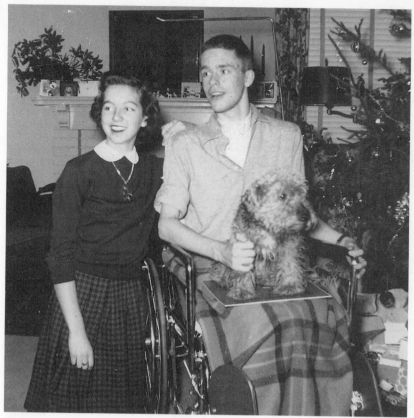

After eight months in hospital, I was allowed home on a Christmas leave. Here I am with my sister Janet by my side and my dog Tigger on my lap. An hour after this photo was taken, a stone unexpectedly began its passage through my kidney and I was returned to the hospital by ambulance with sirens screaming.

silence. I turn the radio on to escape the silence, I always have a symphony on the phonograph. I live in a world with a background of noise. The silence betrays the emptiness of my intellect, the void of my existence. The silence brings the necessity of life and existence before me—truth and purpose.

APRIL 15, WEDNESDAY

I have been talking with a young holy-cross seminarian about Thomas Merton. He agrees with me about several criticisms of

Merton. Merton is extremely emotional, inclined to go off the deep end. His mystical experiences don't quite ring true. At times I get the feeling that he wants to be a saint not only for the love of God but also for the admiration of man. Merton thinks that for grace man must give up the world (almost as Trappists). They may live in the secular world but should rid themselves of newspapers, radio, and T.V. They should stop speaking in their home. I doubt if this quasi-withdrawal is necessary.

Merton feels that speaking, other than praising God is sinful—he doesn't seem to consider writing other than praising God as being sinful. Maybe he does. Anyhow his victory over himself must be praised as must his ability to pass the struggle and victory on to his readers.

I am going out to dinner on Friday! My first meal visit for a year. This is how I will do it. Mother will bring down my clothes and I will put my pants on in bed. Or rather Mother will start them over my braces and I will pull them up. I will then turn on my stomach after having locked the knees of the braces. Mother will drag my legs over the edge of the bed and I will let myself down so that my feet are squarely on the floor. Mother will wheel the chair up behind me and put its brakes on. I will then stand up and ease myself back into the chair. Then I put on my shirt, tie, and jacket and off to the car. Wheel the chair up to the opened car door, extend my braces and pull myself up to a stand on the doorframe with Mother making sure my seat doesn't buckle under me. I pivot and sit on the car seat. And rassle my legs in. At Vera and Larraine's House—where we have been invited to dinner, I reverse the procedure to get out of the car. And Daddy and Mother pull me and chair up their three steps.

It is spring. The air smells deep and good and there are little leaves on the trees and I am waiting for an enema.

Next to my bed there is a bedside table that extends the length of my bed. It is as always piled high with "things." Wherever I go, I seem to collect things in messy profusion. Well there is the 8" Victor radio that Mother has lent me in exchange for my little Sears model. The Victor's tone is better. On top of the radio are 3 little rabbits, gifts of Sister Mary Ellens. You tell me where *she* got them. One of them is wax with a pretty-awful-purple jacket on. The latest *Atlantic* and an old

Popular Mechanics is on the radio too, so is a shaving mirror. There's a book of cowboy songs for the ukulele, the *Iliad* in a new translation, the new *Punch*, Kennan's pessimistic but pretty realistic *American Diplomacy 1900–1950*, a map of Colorado, Carl Sandberg's *Autobiography*, Merton's *Sign of Jonas*, *Bartletts Quotations*, *Madame Bovary* which is boring, a book by Evelyn Waugh whose name I can neither see nor remember, *Crime and Punishment*, a fishing rod and reel and sinker, the telephone, the razor, a bottle of mashed up candy sticks—mashed up because I keep knocking it on the floor, a knife and a stale half eaten cookie. I keep meaning to throw that cookie away.

Today Mother wheeled me up to Pennsylvania Avenue to a bookstore—first one I've been to, since 1952. It is a 3 block walk. I don't like being out in public like that. I am still too sensitive—although I don't know why I am. People don't stare—and I wouldn't mind much if they did. I think it is just my pride. I am unhappy seeing people doing what I can't and I imagine them saying "he doesn't amount to much, he can't even walk, don't look at him." Which is just my old stupid pride—I was just as unhappy watching Joe swim or living with Thomas the strong. It was a problem easier to overcome back in those days. Its importance and difficulty of solution has increased a 100 fold since I've had polio. "Doesn't amount to much"—I'll show them.

All my thought and concentration on the true values of my life, on my aims, on what constitutes happiness shatter when I sally forth into the world in my wheelchair. I forget myself when I see young men of large muscle doing hard jobs, and kids riding bicycles: I think of myself with pity. The last thing in the world I should do.

In short the reason I dislike going out into public is not because of what other people will do or think. It is the depression it throws me into. My thoughts become disoriented.

As Mother was huffing and puffing me up a hill, we passed a little girl of 4 or 5. The little girl crossed herself as we passed. She crossed herself. It was a shock to me. She said a prayer that she wouldn't be like me. Didn't she know how blessed I was. A loving and generous Mother and Father and sister, devoted. Friends, real friends all over the world. A disease in which the worst is over and done with—as compared to those with Muscular Dystrophy or Cancer. And the experience of having suffered pain and torture with the realignment

of values pain and continued torture always brings. I am lucky and
that little girl didn't know.

I bought Franz Kafka's, a neurotic if ever there was one, short stories and Robert Benchley's last book and this week's *Saturday Review*.

APRIL 16, THURSDAY

Inexpressibly beautiful is Bizet's "In the Depths of the Temple" from
the Pearl Fishers (Jussi Bjoerling and Robert Merrill). The voices
blend into something almost unworldly in its beauty. It affects me in
much the way Prokofief's 2nd violin concerto 2nd movement does. It
tears at me. I am careful not to play them too often for then they will
become familiar and common and will lose much of their beauty
for me. For it is transient. Oh for something of permanence—music
of beauty always, art, sculpture truly beautiful and lasting. Such are
nonexistent for they are made by imperfect man and the imperfect
cannot hope to make the perfect. In the same manner inabsolute man
can neither make nor even find by himself an absolute. [Portion of
journal omitted.] For perfection you must look to the mountains, the
desert, to the breeze laden with newness and spring that just came
thru this old and sterile hospital room.

I am going down to Warm Springs on May 5th—just 5 days short
of a year I will have been in hospitals. I told the doctors when I
entered that I couldn't possibly stay more than 3 or 4 days—"Term
paper due that I've hardly started, finals coming, got to get ready for
my Greenland expedition." Since then, I've spent 6 weeks in a respirator; 3 months with a catheter, 3 attacks of cistitis; months of muscle stretching including quadriceps and hamstrings; an operation
for the removal of a bladder stone an inch in diameter; one to remove
a kidney stone that had moved down into the ureter, after an unsuc-
cessful cistoscopy had failed to get it; a breast tumor removed; an
operation at the beginning to install a traceatomy and one last month
to remove it after 10 months of use.

A young man of about my age in white shirt, collar open, sleeves
rolled, with hands in pocket, body relaxed waiting to cross street on
spring evening. His head is up smelling the greatness of being alive on
a spring evening, waiting to cross the street. Of being free and being
able to breathe deeply on a spring evening.

I too can breathe deep but there is no more running with my head back, on the beach, in the spring at night. No more. My running will be done by others.

First outside engagement since illness—dinner at Vera Murphy's and Larraine Davis'. Vera put butter on my plate instead of letting me doing it. She was quite unconscious of it I'm sure. (I sorta like to do what I *can* do.) Evening went fine.

APRIL 20

[Portion of journal omitted.]

My going down to Warm Springs will give my family—especially Mother—a much needed but unadmitted rest. They have been really attentive and loyal. I must gain independence, for their sake as well as mine. I cannot live my life sponging off and being waited on by my parents. And that is that. I must step up my writing, sell some stuff.

[Portion of journal omitted.]

APRIL 21

[Written in pencil] Can't find my pen—darn.

I saw myself today with the help of Jake the orderly and Brother Anthony the Trappist. Jake had some dirty pictures which he brought to show me. They greatly excited my body to the distress (put on or real?) of my brain. Brother Anthony had me play my LP record of the Gregorian Chants and told me a little of the abstinence, rigours, and discipline of monastic life. And the temptations. (The most difficult part of all for me.) This stimulated my brain fully as much as Jake's pictures did my body. But that I could control the body. I could if I knew with a certainty *how* I wanted it controlled. But I don't. I don't seem to have adopted any moral law as my own—cannot bring myself to believe I have found the absolute ethical code. I seem to follow a pragmatic sort of role that if no harm is done to anyone then it is OK. Although I'll admit I am not a judge worthy enough to judge anyone or anything. This is nothing but a comprimize and sidestepping. And chicken.

[Portion of journal is omitted.]

APRIL 23

Adam must have been a real jerk said Brother Anthony.

I am depressed. My new corset doesn't fit me the way I would like—in spite of all its buckles and straps and shoe strings. The two stays stick out in back and I bulge in front. I'm so thin now that I'm hardly here at all but yet that corset gets me bulging. It's getting harder and harder for me to be myself what with all the contraptions they keep harnessing me with. My body is funny enough looking as it is now.

APRIL 24

Doctor agrees with me, corset is being fixed.

APRIL 27

Boy I was depressed, too. It seems as though, before every spurt in body and muscle power that I take, there is a period of depression. When you hit bottom, the only way to go is up. To be trite about it.

It is around six o'clock now and the weather reminds me of the evening of late spring of my year at Tech. There was hate, envy, and jealousy enough for everyone. But there was even more fun and many calm peaceful moments (for me at least) made all the more memorable by the background of distrust and of nervousness, hurry, and tension. On those spring evenings, with the sun lighting the world with slanting rays, the dome of MIT dark and black against the sunset, then it was wonderful. To leave the institute driving fast in Baylis' Ford, looking back at the receding dome, antennae, wire gate, thinking of the summer and how it would be to leave for good. Passing the Diner, pretending it was any roadside diner on the way West. For the West was mountains and desert and they were heaven (Remember Mesa Verde, the knife edge, the distance and Shiprock?) Crossing the railroad spur—looking for Union Pacific and D&RG cars—for just the essence of space and freedom that might have stuck to them. Imagining that we were leaving for good yet knowing that we would end up at the Honey Bee Bar and Restaurant, as usual—

pushing our way thru the drunks and the smoke back to our table, their croquettes and stuffiness. Their New England Plate miraculously changed into Pot Roast by a change of the sauce. Their lemon pies with the rubbery mirangue that fought back. Back thru the mellowed emptied Cambridge streets past the empty silent factories— dreary with generations of dreariness, with all the dullness and plainess that is man made. And yet saved from boredom by the ever newness of spring and the newness of our minds—not yet molded by the dullness and boredom. Freedom and space, the promise of the West, of summer, of independence and all that is glorious.

[Portion of journal omitted.]

April 28

[Portion of journal omitted.]

I would like to write about kind fat little old Miss Glacken and her Aunt Ellen. Miss Glacken wears her hair in a square cut, is at least 60 and has nursed at Providence all her life. She was raised by her aunt, she loves her aunt who is now 89 and senile. Aunt Ellen is in the hospital here with a broken leg at $15 a day. She needs nurses around the clock but Miss Glacken only earns $12 a day. But Aunt Ellen carries on, cries with a bellow like a bull's and asks continually for her niece Mary—who is on another case to make ends meet. Shiny tears form in Mary's eyes when she hears of the carrying-on's of her Aunt for her Aunt was a wonderful, kind, intelligent woman and she loves her. And the hospital says Aunt Ellen can't stay if she carries on and she does; and Mary can't work if she is home with a broken leg.

May 1 or April 30

"April in Portugal" on the radio from the Midwest. In an empty hospital room, alone finally. Dampness of a spring rain outside. Alone and happy. I heard the song once before—it was about 3 a.m. and I was the only one in the stillness of the night, the world Asleep.

"In the depths of the temple" Bizet is of religious significance to me—it seems supreme, unearthly beauty, and I think beauty true is truth and truth must be religion.

WARM SPRINGS

At Warm Springs, I learned the tricks of the trade in physical rehabilitation: getting in and out of a car, transferring from the chair to the toilet, dragging and pivoting myself out of a bathtub. I was also learning something about how to face living with my disability in the years ahead. Although it would be a very long time before I was able to understand (let alone write about) my intense feelings about what had happened to me, I did try.

I LEFT PROVIDENCE HOSPITAL in the spring of 1953, fully a year after the onset of my illness. It had become my home. I loved the old ramshackle hospital built by the Sisters of Charity just after the Civil War. It had high ceilings, wide corridors, and large patient rooms. Mine was the largest, with a bay window which caught the brilliant morning sunshine. Sick bishops kept trying to pull rank and bump me from my room, but the Sisters of Charity stood by me and I retained possession. I remember the Archbishop of Washington had heart disease. He was in a smaller room across the hall. He very much wanted my room but, poor man, he died before he could get it.

The Sisters, the nurses, the doctors, and the cleaning staff had become my friends, and I was loathe to let them go. I had developed a comfortable *modus vivendi* at Providence; it was a closed, safe, little world. I was most reluctant to leave its safety.

I had been accepted for rehabilitation at the Georgia Warm Springs Foundation in Warm Springs, Georgia. I did not want to go. In the hospital with my private duty nurses, my private room, and the severity of my paralysis, I was special. I did not think of myself as being crippled, and I did not want to associate with "cripples." I did not want to be around other paralyzed people.

Warm Springs was a much sought-after place. Polios from across the country applied for entrance, but beds were limited. It took substantial string-pulling on my father's part to get me in. He asked FDR, Jr., to help. So FDR, Jr., asked his mother, Eleanor Roosevelt, to call on my behalf. She did and I was accepted—so now I had to go.

There I was, flying to Georgia. I had my long leg braces on, my backbrace/corset on. I was wearing pressed pants, tweed sport coat, shirt, and tie. In those days, seriously disabled people did not often fly. For that matter, they did not often travel. There were no provisions for the disabled on trains, buses or planes. Wheelchair-accessible hotels were few and far between.

I was paralyzed, not just by polio but by fear—fear of how helpless I would be at Warm Springs, fear at being out in public, fear that I might have to urinate during the flight. There was considerable hassle getting me aboard the aircraft with a forklift. My bulky wheelchair would not fit down the aisle. The airline officials did not know how to carry me, but they were willing, and we did our best. Newspaper photographers were there to record the event. That first trip as a disabled person was a nightmare—and I have the photographs to prove it.

As it turned out, Warms Springs was the best thing ever to happen to me. The difference between life as a patient in the old hospital and rehabilitation at the beautiful resort, deep in the Georgia pines, was as great as the difference between Kansas and Oz.

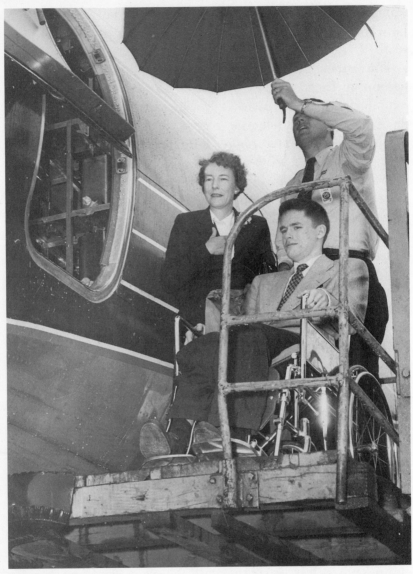

Here I am with my mother on my way to Warm Springs. Note my coat and tie—we were more formal in those days. Mother's concerned look expresses her fear of heights.

There was a soft-spoken elegance about Warm Springs in 1953. An hour-and-a-half from Atlanta, the paved road ended before it reached Warm Springs. The rehabilitation center, known as the Georgia Warm Springs Foundation, was located in the gently rolling hill country in the west of the state.

Founded in the 1920s by Franklin Delano Roosevelt and his fellow polios, the Foundation had a worldwide reputation by the time I arrived in the 1950s. There were patients from all over the 48 states, from Europe and Latin America. The Foundation was cosmopolitan, the little town of Warm Springs was not. Yet the town had always welcomed the polio patients and their families.

The town of Warm Springs and Meriwether County had changed little over the decades. Life there was slow, sleepy and very poor. Back then, the races were strictly segregated. We understood that the Ku Klux Klan was active, but on the campus, we saw nothing of that. Most of the townsfolk worked for the Foundation in one capacity or another. Whether white or black, they were unfailingly kind, cheerful and, as I say, slow. This gave an extraordinary laid-back feeling to the place.

Unlike rehabilitation centers of today, patients stayed a long time at Warm Springs. The average polio would remain at the Foundation for six, eight, ten months, or more. In addition, he or she would return each year for a "checkup" of a week or two. Polio families had built cottages in the woods around the Foundation. Some of them lived in Warm Springs year round; others used their places for vacations. The result was that, in the 1940s and 1950s, there was always an active social life of people coming and going.

The good thing about polio is that, after the acute stage has passed, the patient begins to improve and regain muscle power. This recovery process lasts at least a year or two. There was a high, positive morale at Warm Springs, in part because we were all measurably getting better, month by month.

As the Foundation grounds were self-contained and far from anywhere, the atmosphere was rather like a cruise ship on a long voyage. The place was beautiful and the food was excellent, served in a proper dining room by white-jacketed waiters. Patients and staff came to know each other, lifelong friendships were formed. People fell in love and had affairs. There was always something going on: amateur theatricals, bridge tournaments, visiting celebrities. There was much laughter and gossip.

For me, the experience was very important. Before Warm Springs, I had feared that I would be forced to lead the life of a lonely cripple. At Warm Springs, I found that I could have fun again. Just because I used a wheelchair did not mean I was unable to do things, go places, exert my personality, stretch my intelligence, or use my sex appeal. The Foundation was like a halfway house where I learned how to be me in a wheelchair. For this I am very grateful.

The county was dry; no liquor was allowed. The Foundation had a strict rule: anyone caught drinking on campus was discharged and sent home. In addition, my doctors told me I must not smoke because my lungs were so very weak. Until Warm Springs, no one had ever told me I could not drink or smoke. In point of fact, I had never done either, nor had I any interest in doing so. But at Warm Springs, I was *ordered* not to. I react badly to authority. My character is such that, if someone tells me I must not do something, I feel compelled to do it. This was the case with alcohol and tobacco.

I learned to drink moonshine—and later Scotch—at Warm Springs and I still drink Scotch. I began smoking at Warm Springs, and I smoked a pack or two a day for more than ten years, a bad and dangerous habit. They said *don't*, so I *did*.

My Warm Springs Journal

Here are a few entries from my journal. They give a sense of what Warm Springs was like in the 1950s.

May 2

8 months to the day—I left Providence yesterday.

May 5

I am now in Warm Springs. I was home Friday, Saturday, Sunday, and Monday. And now I am here. Georgia is all red clay. It has been raining the last week they tell me. Anyhow it looks as though all of Georgia is washing away into Florida. Most of the houses along the highway are unpainted and propped up on bricks.

MAY 8

I'm not doing very well with my journal—living with three room-mates is not conducive to classic writing. Right now there are six people in here—difficult, hard to think.

A boy left for home today with his folks. He has been here 8 months. He wears a corset, full leg braces, and has tricep crutches. A good-looking guy of 19 with a serious, worried face. His parents have been here the last 4 days, learning how to continue their son's therapy. His mother is a pretty, intelligent Southern lady, his father a staunch family man. They are bright, cheerful when their son is around, and nervous. When he isn't near, their attitudes change as do their faces. They love their son, their only son, and he is crippled badly, almost terribly. He was to go to college, his father's pride was unbounded, all was happiness—before polio. And now they feel that the world has shattered and is lying about them in pieces. They haven't yet learned how to pick up the pieces, how to slowly rebuild their world. (They will but it will take time.) There is sadness in his mother's eyes, and pride—pride that her boy is alive. He himself is depressed and this depression acts to increase the anxiety and nervousness of his parents. *Their* anxiety just increases the depression of their son.

I saw the mother learning how to walk her son.

More about above, later. They tell me that I have no muscles from my shoulders down. None. None. There is more to life than muscles. There must be.

MAY 9 SATURDAY

Boy, are there a lot of interesting, nice type, worried looking people around here. On the porch now there is a family of five. They are coarse, rugged-looking people—probably from the hills. Here to see their son (or daughter), they have been waiting on the porch. Pa has on overalls—the real kind with shoulder straps and copper buckles. His stomach protrudes a little and he has on rimless glasses. He is trying to be genial with wide, friendly smiles as the patients wheel by in their chairs. His nose is long and his shoes are pointed with air vents. His wife is dressed in her best. Her dress is a bright purple—the color spilled purple ink that has dried. It has yarn tassles hanging all over it. She also has on an Easter-egg pink jacket—part of a suit, probably from Ward's. She looks as though she's dressed to be cheerful, to raise the spirits of someone, to keep up her own. Her face is worn with time; there is tragedy in her eyes. The sister is pregnant but has no maternity dress. She is used to pregnancy. They all are lined up against the wall, staring into the green-shaded space. They don't say anything. Evidently, Southern folk from the hills don't say much. Anyhow, this family says nothing. Just stare into space. Their clothes are different but their emotions aren't.

FEBRUARY 28, 1954   WASHINGTON

It has been almost a year since I last wrote in this journal. It hardly seems so. The progress I have made in my return to life or in my adjustment to paralysis has been great, but there is much ground still left to cover. Last May—a year after the onset of my polio—I was unable to care for myself in any way. During my 8 months I was taught physical independence. An ability to take care of one's self by one's self is one of the greatest and dearest gifts man has. Its loss is one of man's greatest tragedies. For if you require the help of some-one else to put your shirt on, you lose your personal identity, your physical oneness during that period of time that the act is taking place. You cease to be you; you become a part of someone else in that instant of assistance. And that is why my heart bleeds when I see someone who is completely helpless, even if he has a loving wife or mother to help him. Perhaps even more so, for he becomes so much more firmly bound, tightly laced to their lives by his depen-dence. His whole existence must be spent in struggling to assert his ego, his soul, his being. And that is why sometimes, when I'm off my guard, I feel sorry for myself. Sorry that I can't run across a lawn or walk the lakeshore by myself. There's the crux—by myself. I resent always being accompanied, even if by friends and family—or maybe especially by my family.

REHABILITATION

This is an excerpt from my book, FDR's Spendid Deception.* *It describes the rehabilitation process developed at Warm Springs. This is the treatment I received during the nine months I was at the Georgia Warm Springs Foundation.*

BY THE LATE 1920S, the policies and procedures followed by the Georgia Warm Springs Foundation had been firmly established. Over the next 30 years, new buildings would be constructed, the rehabilitation equipment would become more sophisticated, and treatment policy would evolve. Nevertheless, the basics remained unchanged.

What Roosevelt conceived at Warm Springs seems, on reflection, to be both sensible and obvious, but it was, in fact, revolutionary. So far as rehabilitation practice is concerned, Roosevelt grasped certain principles intuitively; his actions and decisions were based upon these prin-

---

*Vandamere Press, Arlington, VA, 1995.

ciples, even though they had not yet been formalized into words or placed within the context of an organized, philosophical structure. At Warm Springs, Roosevelt and his associates were busy *doing* rehabilitation. As a result, they discovered various principles, and these were later incorporated into a coherent theory of rehabilitation.

This intuitive understanding of a problem and its solution, this development of the principle of the solution in concert with the practical application of the solution, was the method Roosevelt would use later in the New Deal.

From the first, Roosevelt seemed to understand that rehabilitation of the polio patient was a social problem with medical aspects. It was not a medical problem with social aspects, as previous American treatment efforts had assumed. Most modern hospitals and rehabilitation centers give lip service to this concept, but, even now, remarkably few seem willing to act upon it.

Patients came to Warm Springs after the acute stage of their illness, sometimes years after. They were often in a state of mind bordering on shell shock. They were hurt and grieving still from the loss of use of their paralyzed limbs. They felt helpless and angry as a result of the hospital treatment they had received. The impact of a severe hospital regime upon the paralyzed person often causes a regression into infantile behavior. Responsibility for eating, urinating, and bowel movements, for getting up and going to bed, are removed from the patient and exercised by medical authority, assuming the role of a strict parent. The good patient, like a good child, does what he is told. Such a patient is rewarded for his dependent behavior; the rebel is punished. Obviously, this procedure is not rehabilitative; it is, in fact, debilitative.

Such treatment was universal when Roosevelt began Warm Springs. It produced anger and confusion, and it was particularly difficult for teenagers. Adolescents are in the process of separating from their families and parents. They have not yet established themselves as fully-functioning, self-reliant adults. Typical hospital routines complicated or blocked these efforts. Teenagers are particularly vulnerable in another way. During the adolescent years, there is generally great concern about body development as the frame develops and sexual characteristics mature. The adolescent child is particularly sensitive to, and self-conscious about, body changes. Severe paralysis of the adolescent child can have a catastrophic psychological impact, destroying concepts of self-worth, raising vast self-doubt.

The Warm Springs experience had an immediate impact upon such shell-shocked patients. For the long-term patient who had come from the grim Victorian hospitals, the effect was sometimes quite stunning. The Warm Springs setting was physically of great beauty: flowers everywhere, manicured lawns, tall green pines, and blue skies. Rooms were bright and sunny; the food was excellent; help was readily available; and the importance of fun was both appreciated and cultivated.

The patient realized from the first that Warm Springs was quite different. This difference produced a change of attitude in him or her—a positive change.

Under Roosevelt's direction, the medical treatment at Warm Springs was divided into segments: the polio patient would receive the physical therapy treatments necessary to maximize muscle recovery and would learn the techniques necessary to allow functioning in society to the maximum extent possible.

The physical therapy provided at Warm Springs was always of excellent quality. The staff was highly competent. As the Foundation's reputation grew, therapists from across the country sought admission to its training programs. The brace shop at Warm Springs acquired a nationwide reputation for excellence and innovation. Warm Springs innovated water treatment techniques and developed numerous creative and useful prosthetic devices. Many professional articles by staff members on various aspects of this treatment were published in medical journals.

From the first, Warm Springs placed unusual emphasis on functional training. This was quite new. Patients at Warm Springs took part in classes in which they learned how to make use of whatever muscles were available to them so as to get in and out of bathtubs, on and off toilets, in and out of cars, and how to perform the routine tasks of day-to-day living. The class concept was important. Patients with similar degrees and kinds of paralysis worked together. They gave each other suggestions and ideas and, equally important, they gave each other encouragement and support. These classes were occasions of much laughter. Severe paralysis often causes absurd predicaments, which can be very funny. It was a warm and cheerful experience to work with others to overcome these problems.

For a generation, Warm Springs was a community of the handicapped. A permanent population of polios came to live at the Foundation or nearby. Many of these people worked at the Foundation as officials, staff people, and teachers. In 1930, there were eight polios on the rehabilitation staff. Other resident polios were well-to-do people who found life comfortable and protective at Warm Springs and simply decided to stay. Still others came down for the winter season from their homes in the North. The presence of these people helped both the functional training and the social aspects of the Warm Springs treatment.

Leaders of the functional training classes would invite the older resident polios to demonstrate their techniques—the tricks and methods they had devised to perform the daily tasks of life with partially paralyzed muscles. This was of benefit to the new patients in practical terms, but also in psychological terms more difficult to describe and define. New polios saw the old polios as persons with a paralysis pattern similar to their own, living a normal life, functioning as productive human beings. The value of such an example was enormous.

At Warm Springs, social life served a purpose greater than simple morale building. It provided a way for polio patients to relearn their social skills. Warm Springs provided an opportunity to meet people, undertake joint activities, make friends, date, fall in love. The whole range of normal social activities went on at Warm Springs, much the way it does elsewhere in the world. New patients were welcomed into the group. Their handicap did not isolate them from the norm; it *was* the norm. The parties, dinners, and activities at Warm Springs gave new patients the opportunity to exercise the skills, traits, and habits they developed and used in interpersonal contact before their illness. And, of course, in most cases, the patients found that people responded in much the way they had before the illness. He or she was as attractive, as witty, and had the same positive and negative traits as before. This realization was helpful in the reconstruction of self-image.

At Warm Springs, parties were as important to rehabilitation as the treatment table or the walking court. The Foundation was a microcosmos, a protected halfway house. The social practice available in this protected environment gave patients a confidence that would allow them to move more easily in the world of the able-bodied upon their return to their home environments.

Life at Warm Springs was never puritanical. The gray pall of institutional life never threatened the Foundation. Meals were important and festive. The tables were set with good china and linen napkins and tablecloths. The food was fresh, well cooked, and served by well-trained waiters in dinner jackets. Places at table were reserved, the makeup of the table at dinner carefully planned. There were bridge tournaments and poker games, classes, movies, excursions, amateur theatricals, and visiting professional artists. There were private dinners, cocktail parties in the cottages, and, as always with the Roosevelts, picnics. Many of these activities were spontaneous; none was forced. As at Greenbrier, White Sulphur Springs, or Saratoga in season, Warm Springs was a cheerful, active, lovely resort in the country. And, of course, during the 12 years when FDR was in the White House, it was a place of great glamour and excitement.

In the United States, polio struck most heavily at teenagers. The youthful patient population at Warm Springs added to its vitality. Roosevelt is said to have felt strongly that these young people needed to be encouraged, not only in their social life, but also in their sexual life. He hired local high school boys, he called them "push boys"— and they were available at all hours to push the patients in wheelchairs where they might wish to go. Push boys were not in short supply—one was almost always within earshot. They were to be used not simply to go to and from treatment, but to the coffee shop, post office, the movie theater—wherever the patient might wish to go. From a local girls' college, Roosevelt obtained the services of eight girls, majoring in physical science. These were employed as assistant physical therapists. In a very tangible sense, the presence of these young women and men interacting with the patients helped keep Warm Springs a lively place. There was flirting, falling in love, sexual hanky-panky—and much gossip about it all.

In 1980, at a meeting in Washington called to consider the disposition of the Warm Springs property, Anne Irwin Bray, whose father had been medical director, was reunited with Toi Bachelder, herself a Warm Springs polio, who had served as a secretary to President Roosevelt. As they began to exchange stories of the FDR days, their memories flooded in upon them.

"Oh Toi," said Anne, *"wasn't it fun!"*

MRS. ROOSEVELT VISITS WARM SPRINGS

Warm Springs patients published a small mimeographed magazine on a biweekly basis. When FDR was still alive, a copy would go directly to the president's desk in the oval office. He was a faithful reader. By the time I was the editor, FDR was no longer alive, but the journal was still a staple of Warm Springs life.

Here is a story I wrote when Mrs. Roosevelt came to visit. I remember the scene clearly. Georgia Hall is a large, long room. It was absolutely jammed that day. People were standing on their long leg braces and crutches; others were using wheelchairs, and still others were lying on wheeled gurneys. The noise and hubble-bubble were exceptional. Reporters, photographers and those big old television cameras added to the excitement. It could not have been easy to confront such a throng of disabled people but Mrs. R. had toured the battlefields of the South Pacific and addressed a crowd of a million people in India. She was an old pro and, as soon as she started talking, she made us feel at ease.

Apparently Mrs. Roosevelt told the Warm Springs manager that she would like to meet me. I was duly located and presented to the former

First Lady. She reminded me exactly of my grandmother: she walked fast, had sensible shoes, and was quick to notice everything. She held in her hand a small, worn spiral notebook which had my name along with two or thee others written in pencil. She explained to me that she had told her son she would look me up and see how I was doing. She asked me several questions about my treatment and actually made notes in her book. When she returned to Hyde Park, she called my parents to give them a report on my progress. They were as surprised as they were grateful for her call.
The following week, for a split second or two, I was in the newsreels!

MRS. ROOSEVELT VISITS WARM SPRINGS*

Mrs. Franklin D. Roosevelt, wife of the founder of the Foundation, visited Warm Springs last Wednesday, September 30. She was in the area for only half a day, but in that time she visited the Little White House, the Foundation, and Dowdell's Knob, site of the proposed multimillion dollar Hall of History.

The first official notice of her visit that the patients received was an announcement at Wednesday lunch that anyone interested in seeing Mrs. Roosevelt should be in Georgia Hall by three o'clock.

At three, the Hall was jammed. Wheelchairs and stretchers, patients at three o'clock walking class which was being held inside because of the rain, and people watching the World Series were all awaiting Mrs. Roosevelt. She arrived at 3:30 in a Cadillac limousine, escorted by Charles F. Palmer of Atlanta. She was greeted at the door by Mr. Fred Botts, GWSF Director of Admissions and longtime friend of the Roosevelts.

With a smile on her face and with the kind of courage Daniel must have had to face the lions, she turned and entered the Hall jammed with expectant patients. She was introduced to the assembled by Mr. Botts, who called her "one of the great women of the world." She stood before the group straight and tall, for she is a large woman; a maroon faille blouse, a gray skirt, and sensible black oxfords were her

---

*First published, *Warm Springs News*, October, 1953

dress. She looked for all the world like someone's grandmother, as indeed she is. She spoke to the patients.

"I am very happy to come to Warm Springs and see all the improvements that have been made," said Mrs. Roosevelt. "It's wonderful to see the work my husband started here and which did him so much good going on to help other people find life more interesting and livable. I hope you all will hold to the feeling that life is worth living and that you are making a contribution to the United States. For what goes on here offers the whole world something important."

She said that she had been asked all over the world about the treatment and research going on at Warm Springs. The Foundation and each and every patient are making "an important contribution" to the care of treatment of polio, she added.

Mrs. Hazel Stephens, Director of Functional Training, conducted Mrs. Roosevelt on a tour of the new building, Roosevelt Hall. The building, dedicated last fall by Basil O'Connor, director of the National Foundation of Infantile Paralysis, will be devoted largely to Functional Training and Occupational Therapy. Mrs. Roosevelt also visited the infirmary and treatment pool.

Under the glare of kleig lights and amid the whir of newsreel cameras, she said her good-byes; and, less than 40 minutes after her arrival, she was off, on her way back to Atlanta and her speaking tour.

My Brother

I wrote this piece, "My Brother," in 1955, a year after I left Rehab. Never published until now, it is an account of a patient who was at Warm Springs when I was there. In the story, I called him Floyd, but his real name was Leroy. I see now that I projected on poor Leroy my own fears about disability and the limitation it imposes. This was the first of several pieces I have written in which I used someone else as a vehicle to express emotions about myself—emotions I was unable to confront directly.

WARM SPRINGS WAS, of course, founded by Franklin Roosevelt who caught polio in the 1920s. It was a newspaper article describing the wonder-working qualities of the natural springs that first brought the place to his attention.

When he arrived he found several other polios taking the baths. Warm Springs was, and is, a pleasant little resort in the Georgia hills. Since antebellum days, it has been a summer resort for the Atlanta aristocracy. Roosevelt soon found, as did the other polios, that the springs were not in the least wonder-working, but they also found that the daily exercises in the pool were helpful for strengthening weakened muscles. The water, by removing the enervating pull of gravity, gave muscles too weak to exercise against gravity a chance to slowly gain power through gentle, buoyant movement.

As more polios gathered, learning of the springs by word of mouth, Roosevelt and the original old-timers formed the Georgia Warm Springs Foundation. Funds were accumulated and soon there was an active group of doctors, therapists, and brace-makers established on the Foundation.

Although Warm Springs has grown to the point where there are always over a hundred polios convalescing, it has never lost its pleasant resort-like atmosphere. The Georgia sun is always warm, the tall Georgia pines are still stately and soothing. Life is slow and comfortable in the manner that is traditional in the deep South.

There are cocktail parties and dinners, expeditions to Atlanta and picnics on Pine Mountain. These are the events that give the pleasure of expectancy to the slowly moving days. The patients, the therapists, the doctors and all their families take part in this slightly smug, yet always comforting, life.

The President is no longer present at the parties or the Thanksgiving banquet, but the spirit, the friendliness, and the secluded content are still there, still part of Warm Springs.

This spirit is what makes Warm Springs so attractive to convalescing polios who have spent all too many months in the sterility of hospital wards. They are overjoyed at finding themselves part of a functioning normal-like society again.

The new patient, surrounded by many in the same situation and some in a worse situation, casts off his self-pity or soon has it forcibly torn from him by his neighbors, who will tolerate practically anything but pity or despair. The pity of others, the self-pity you feel yourself feel when your body is helpless, combine in despair; overcoming this pity is the most difficult struggle of all. This is a struggle that all polios must make, at one time or another, if they are to recover. It must be faced, but not now, not here on the Foundation.

And so underneath this pleasant and cheerful spirit runs a current of uncertainty, of uneasiness. "You don't adjust at Warm

Springs," says the Foundation psychologist. "That comes afterwards, when you leave. Our job is to strengthen you—physically and mentally, for the adjustment that is to come." The patients sense this; they know within themselves that they dread this readjustment, this battle for normalcy that must come. Their families and their therapists feel it too. It is always there. So they have parties and do mad things, drink moonshine, and go to the movies. The younger patients have love affairs; the older patients gossip about them. The casual visitor is amazed at the carefree fun. The returning checkup patient understands it.

I arrived at Warm Springs in May of 1953 and soon found myself in a happy group, in love off and on, working on the paper, and laughing more than I ever had or ever have since that time. If sometimes when I was alone, I found myself wondering what I could possibly make of my future, it wasn't hard to find a bridge game or a coffee group and push the future into the distant indefinite.

Social life centered around dinner. The people who sat at your table were your particular friends, and the protocol of table arrangements was as complex as the seating of the Windsors at a benefit banquet. At my table there was Andrea Doré, a beautiful dark haired girl from New Orleans, the first real Southern belle I had ever known. She expected all men to wait on her, to answer her slightest whim; most men were only too happy to oblige. I was desperately in love with her, or so I thought.

Lorenzo Morris, of New York and Jacksonville, had come down with polio during his junior year at Yale. He was extraordinarily adept at smuggling Scotch onto the Foundation.

Maggie Clark was our fourth. She had caught polio in Madrid where she was a member of the Foreign Service. Her distinction was having lived three years in Madrid without ever once missing a bullfight or ever once visiting the Prado.

It was at dinner one night that I first heard of Floyd.

"Have you seen him yet?" Andrea asked.

"Seen who?" we all replied.

"The little boy from Arkansas." She paused, "He's just too horrible. He's twisted and . . ." She had her hands on the arms of her wheelchair holding on; her face was dull and without light. It was this, I think, that stopped our usual four-way conversation. As her voice trailed off, I think we all felt ourselves being propelled forward, faster than we wanted.

The Warm Springs dining room is a large room with at least 50 tables. It is furnished with taste, painted a Williamsburg green, with a portrait of President Roosevelt hanging on the far wall.

All the waiters are blacks, dressed in white coats; the headwaiter is always in a tuxedo. Although the atmosphere is neither formal nor stiff, it is true that everyone makes a point of dressing up for dinner.

It wasn't more than a minute or so after Andrea had finished talking that Floyd rolled into the dining room. He turned down our aisle, unseen by the busy headwaiter. We pretended not to notice him— we who knew what it must be like for him.

Let me describe him as he wheeled down the aisle toward us. He was as shocking as Andrea had said. He was obviously not a new polio; he had been crippled for many years. It is only over a long period of years—during the growing childhood of a polio—that deformities may appear. These are caused by muscle weakness on one side of the body that is overbalanced by strength on the other. Severely unbalanced muscle power is very dangerous for a growing child.

Floyd could not have been more than 17 years old. His face was a good one; it had character. Later when I had talked with him, I was conscious of seeing deeply into his eyes. It was as though another person in another world looked out through Floyd's eyes. This other person lived far away from me and from Floyd, far back into those blue eyes. His hair was blonde and was beautifully combed. Each blonde wave was perfection.

His body, how can I describe it? It was like a mechanical sea monster waving its jointed tentacles—like a tarantula turned upon its back waving its legs. Floyd's back had been badly malformed. It looked to me as though he had had polio since infancy without any medical care at all. This we later found to be true. His spine was bent to such a degree that his rib cage on his left side had fused with his pelvis. He had no waist. His T shirt and blue jeans, faded and ripped, covered a jumble, just a heap of torso. His right shoulder was higher than his head, his left seeming to be completely nonexistent. He wheeled himself with a motion of flinging himself forward, his long and skinny arms jerking out at odd angles, his deformed hands grasping the wheels between the first and third joints of the fingers; his thumbs sticking out paralyzed and useless. His progress was jerky and sporadic.

The headwaiter came up behind Floyd, as he was passing our table. "Let me help you, son," he said, taking hold of the chair.

Floyd's head jerked, "I can do it myself. See if I can't." He sat by himself at the end of the aisle that night.

As I said before, our table pretended not to notice as Floyd went by, and our jokes and games and crazy laughter went on as before. But they were not the same. Occasionally I would glance down at Floyd, eating alone. I wonder how many other of the new polios looked at Floyd that night.

In the lobby after dinner, I asked the Foundation's social worker about Floyd. She had talked to him that afternoon. Floyd was from Arkansas, a poor family in the Ozarks. He had evidently had polio as a baby, but the Arkansas Infantile Paralysis Foundation had found him only a couple of years ago. They had bought him a wheelchair. Until that time he had crawled about on the floor much as a crab would scuttle across the bed of the ocean. This year they had raised enough money to send him here for a consultation on what could be done for him. "And I'm afraid that not much can be done," said Mrs. Freyman, our social worker. "A spine, once it's really deformed, can't be straightened."

"Those hamstrings and quads are so tight they couldn't straighten his legs in a hundred years," said Sarah Vaughn, a therapist. "If only they had caught the kid when he first got sick," they agreed, "if only."

"He doesn't go to school," said Mrs. Freyman. "He doesn't do anything that I can see. He says he likes to sit out under the trees. Says he knows some of the birds and the squirrels. He talks a lot about a brother, the poor guy. He whittles, too. That's all he said."

"If only," we agreed, "if only they had found him earlier."

"My brother goes to school," said Floyd the next morning. I had swallowed my disgust or whatever it was and rolled up to talk to him. I hated myself for feeling this way but I must admit he made me sick to my stomach. "He can read," Floyd said looking at me from behind those eyes of his. He spoke with an exaggerated drawl.

"Isn't that nice," I replied, instinctively using the tone of a kindergarten teacher addressing her charges.

"Yeah, he goes to school. He reads and everything. He takes out girls and really does things to them. He tells me all about it."

Floyd seemed very unsure, and his bravado was that of an unprotected thing. His pride in his brother was held up to me as proof of his own being. It was like watching the helpless flight of a bat exposed to a brilliant searchlight.

He told me that morning about the dirty stories his brother had told him, about how his brother played baseball and hunted, how his Ma never yelled at his brother.

It all made me ill and embarrassed. He was likable—almost pitiably so—and twisted. I think we all pretended he wasn't so. We pretended not to see him. It wasn't that he was deformed or twisted, there were many polios at Warm Springs who were deformed, but there were few who were *so* deformed. And there were none so naked. He stood before us as he was: without defense or wisecracks, no nice clothes, no interesting experiences, his hair meticulously combed, his brother, and that was all.

Floyd was rushed through the incoming process for polios past convalescent stage. He went faster than any I had seen. It was as though even the doctors wanted him over and done with as fast as they could manage it.

The series of necessary X-rays, muscle tests, tightness exams, and doctor's conferences is bewildering enough to any new patient. I can only imagine what it was to Floyd.

We all knew there was nothing that could be done for him. The tests only served to prove this. His spine was badly curved. A spinal fusion or a plaster jacket—the treatments for curvature—are useful only before the spine begins to angle. They can to some degree prevent deformity; they can in no way cure an excessive deformity already present.

His frail legs could be straightened through a series of operations cutting the calcified tendons. But what would this serve? Even with his legs braced and straightened, how could Floyd, his whole trunk fused into shapelessness, hope to walk? Treatments, operations— there was nothing to be done.

Floyd stayed with us only a week. No one talked about him much— for what was there to say? The fun and the gaiety that week seemed pretty forced to me. Someone was present who wasn't playing, who had never had the chance of playing. He sat and watched us through his eyes, an awry grin on his face perhaps, his hair combed always. We tried to talk to him, we tried to be kind, and it was worse. We tried to take him into our game and he was naked before us, he didn't know how to play. We would have given him our game but he did not know how to take it. The safety of the Foundation was no safety to him. The game he did not know how to play, he had already lost.

He never seemed to talk about his polio. The only thing I remember him saying about himself he said in conference with Dr. Bennet, the Medical Director of the Foundation. My therapist, Helen Harkness, was present. Floyd said nothing at all as his X-rays and reports were discussed. Only as the conference was ending, did he say in a low voice, "Last year I could walk real good." Helen tells me that Dr. Bennet snorted with incredulity. It just wasn't so.

Floyd's only conversation was about his brother—his brother who did wonderful things. These were things all boys do, but to Floyd they were wonderful. His love for his brother was everything in his life. Andrea tells me that she once asked him if his brother didn't sometimes take him along so that he could join in doing some of these things. She could see, as soon as she had asked, that the question was unfair.

"He doesn't have time," Floyd told her. "He's got too much to do. But he tells me all about them. You know I reckon he can drink more corn liquor than any guy in the county!"

No one talked to him much—what could one say? But everyone tried to do something for him.

The Foundation teacher taught him to add and subtract and how to count money. They gave him $5.00 of his own when he left. It was the first money he had ever had of his own. His gratefulness was as clear as it was embarrassing. He had no conception of what to do with the money.

He tried to give it to Andrea; he had fallen in love with her. She and Margaret taught him to tell time and bought him an Ingersoll watch. He had never known time other than a little or a lot. A minute was a little, a year a lot. Now he had a clock to count the hours of his life.

The therapists took him over to Manchester and bought him a couple of pairs of jeans and several T-shirts. Lorenzo and I gave him a going-away present of a carton of Lucky Strikes.

All of this was done silently, secretly, almost ashamedly. For what did any of it mean? Why count money when you have none, why count hours when you have none but hours? What *do* you have—a brother?

When he left the Foundation, he told Mrs. Freyman, "I sure wish my brother could meet all you folks. He sure would like you all." It was more thanks than any of us deserved.

It was Mrs. Freyman who, in reading through his records later sent from Arkansas, discovered that Floyd was an only child. He had no brothers. But by then, what with our romances, gossip and game, we were too busy to care.

RETURN TO COLLEGE

In the spring of 1954, I wrote over 40 letters to colleges across the country, seeking one that would be accessible to my wheelchair. I received nothing but turndowns, until purely by serendipity, I found Claremont McKenna College in Claremont, California. I had two happy years at CMC and obtained my American B.A. in June, 1956, only two years delayed by polio.

I had always hoped to attend Oxford University in the United Kingdom. I saw no reason why the wheelchair should stand in my way. Accordingly, I applied for a Rhodes Fellowship. In due course, my application was returned to me, unprocessed.

Cecil Rhodes had specified in his will that his fellowships should go only to men who were "fit in mind and body." I was healthy but paralyzed—did I qualify as "fit"? I learned later that the Rhodes Trust convened a special meeting to debate the question at Rhodes House, Oxford. My application, I later learned, was the first they had ever received from a disabled person. The board, after careful deliberation, decided to sidestep the issue altogether. Instead of ruling on my fitness,

they would return my application as though it had never been
received. I was a "nonapplicant"!

This was a very English sort of rejection. The rejection made me all
the more determined that I would go to Oxford and that I would find
a way to do it. This, of course, was a very American reaction.

I reprint below the essay I wrote for the Rhodes application. I do so
because it illustrates how I was trying to deal with my handicap: I
would let it "enter my life only when it is impossible to keep it out."
This approach, I was to learn over and over, does not work very well.
Such an attitude, in effect, turns your paralyzed body into the enemy
at the gate, lurking about, always seeking a way to betray your plans.

MY LIFE SO FAR

Perhaps the easiest way of explaining myself, my interests, and my
plans would be to begin at the beginning.

I entered the Massachusetts Institute of Technology in the fall of
1950, planning to major in electrical engineering. Because of my
father's occupation—public administration—my family has lived in
various places throughout the United States and, for a year, in Greece.
I grew up in a continual cycle of starting at new schools, making new
friends, and establishing myself, only to begin the process all over
again in a year or two. I wanted permanence.

Books, ideas, and writing are part of my family and my life; but,
by entering M.I.T., I meant to renounce the curiosity and searching
for which they stood.

I was looking for permanence and security. An engineer is an engineer, I thought: a man who knows just what he wants and knows how
to get it.

This may be true, but I soon found that this security was another
name for complacency; and that to achieve it, I would have to sacri-
fice my writing and my books. These were of little importance when
I was with them at home; they became of overwhelming importance
after a year of what seemed the tedious busywork of putting numbers
in formulas.

I was at the Institute on a scholarship, and I did well scholastically, although not outstandingly so.

I worked on the school paper, was elected to its managing board in May, and was destined for the editorship. I took part in various other campus organizations.

My dissatisfaction and inner confusion came to a head in September of my second year. I had been doing a lot of reading, Daedalus' struggling through his lectures on Maxwell's equations, in Joyce's *Portrait of the Artist as a Young Man,* was very like my own. Thomas Wolfe in *Of Time and the River,* pulling volume after volume down from the shelves of Widener, desperately wringing knowledge from them, pointed up the shallowness of my own goal of stolidity.

I read Plato for the first time. Socrates subverted me no less than he did the Athenians. I threw over what was for me, and possibly is for my generation, the principal goal—a nonexistent security. It may seem trite to say that Socrates is responsible for my search for meaning and truth, my determination to make of my life something of true value; but he is.

I left the Institute, and I have never regretted the leaving—especially in the light of my bout with polio.

I entered Haverford to major in writing and government. I wanted a broad education in philosophy, literature, and the humanities.

I was at Haverford but a semester. During that time, I was appointed sports editor of their paper and was told that I would become editor-in-chief the following year. I worked like a fanatic. I worked hard on the paper and harder on my courses, which urged me on to still more reading. I argued late into many nights over truth, reality, and beauty with a zeal that seems now more overwhelming than anything else.

The summer before, I worked on a railroad gang in the Rockies. I lived out by myself, sleeping bag, et al., and had a profitable summer—but a hard one, physically.

In May of my first year at Haverford, I came down with spinal and bulbar polio. I was in an iron lung for six weeks and in hospital for two years.

I learned a lot during these years. I learned not to be afraid of pain; I gained an inkling of what man can bear; I learned how real and valuable friendship is and how invaluable and powerful love can be.

Without the love and faith of my parents, I would not be alive today.

My interest in ideas, my love of books, stood me in great stead. During the months of my convalescence, my parents encouraged, supplied, and, in turn, whetted my interests.

When I returned home from the Warm Springs Rehabilitation Center, I was physically independent, healthy, and in a wheelchair. I still am.

I spent nine months working for Congressman Aspinall of Colorado. This involved writing letters, doing research projects, and condensing speeches. The training I received on the functioning of government was invaluable. The confidence I gained from being out in the world again was equally as valuable.

In September of 1954, I drove my own car across the country to Claremont, California, to enroll at Claremont Men's College.

At present, I am still at C.M.C. I am still reading a great deal and writing a lot. I was made managing editor of the school paper last spring, and this fall was elected president of my dormitory. During the 1954 election campaign, I founded a Young Democrat's group on campus and, with a friend in the spring of that year, organized a weekly Constitutional Study Group.

My months in the hospital gave me time to reform my ambitions and aims.

I decided to let polio enter my life only when it is impossible to keep it out.

I would do what I had planned and worked for, before getting sick, but I would do it without the hysteria of the Haverford days.

I hope to be an author. I am interested in politics and government, and I would like to write in this field. Exactly how, I am not sure: journalism, if possible—perhaps political history or biography—perhaps work in political science theory.

Up until a few years ago, anyone in a wheelchair was relegated, symbolically and actually, to the back-room with the blinds drawn.

The handicapped are as able, intelligent, and willing as the unhandicapped. I feel, however, that it is up to the handicapped to prove this. When a person in a wheelchair does something of worth, he brings honor, not only to himself, but to all other people in wheelchairs. I try always to remember this.

I have wanted to study at Oxford, ever since I made a short visit there in 1948, when returning from Greece.

If I should get the chance to go to Oxford, I would plan my course so as to take maximum advantage of the library and research facilities, the historic tradition and atmosphere, and the emphatic insistence upon disciplined, lucid, and graceful writing.

I would like to work in Modern Greats—the Honour School of Philosophy, Politics, and Economics. Although specializing in politics, I would like to get as broad and deep a background in literature, history, and philosophy as possible.

My college career so far has been a curious odyssey. I have been through a lot; I have made mistakes. But I do not regret a bit of it. I am a better man now than I was in the fall of 1950.

OXFORD LIFE

I did go to Oxford. I went as a Marshall Fellow, a scholarship funded by the British government, for which I was most grateful. I was up at the University for three years, during which time I was the only person using a wheelchair in the entire university.

OXFORD LIFE FOR A PERSON in a wheelchair was strange indeed. I was there from 1956 to 1959. The university consists of 35 individual colleges. My college was Trinity. It was the only college to have a bedroom, bathroom, dining room and chapel on the ground floor; hence, it was the only college accessible to a wheelchair.

Trinity traditionally draws its students from the old country Whig aristocracy. It is a Stuart college in that it refused to recognize William and Mary's claim to the throne in the Glorious Revolution of 1688. The front gates were closed and padlocked never to be opened again until a Stuart is restored to the monarchy. The gates are now welded shut.

Trinity was one ot the few colleges left at Oxford to maintain its aristocratic standards. It still retained the prewar tradition of pro-

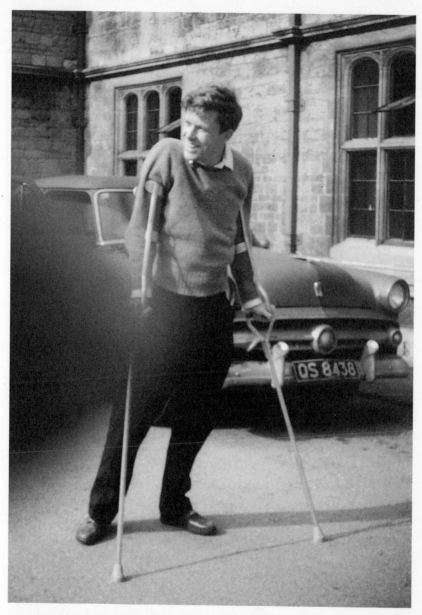

Although I lack the strength to move my legs, I can stand like this indefinitely. Standing gives me a psychological boost—it reminds me that I am a tall man. Above, I am standing on my braces and crutches beside my hand-controlled car in front of my rooms at Trinity College, Oxford.

viding men servants ("scouts") for its students. This was fine by me. My scout was named Spanner, and I could not have survived the English winters without his help.

I had two rooms in college, a living room and a bedroom. There was a fireplace in the living room. There was no heat whatsoever in the bedroom. Spanner would arrive early every morning. He would clean up the living room and stoke up the coal fire. When it was going well, he would wake me, bringing me my mail in bed. I would jump out of bed quickly in the cold, and dress before the fire in the living room. By then, Spanner would have brought a teakettle of hot water to the washstand. I would wash my face and hands, shave, leaving it for Spanner to dump my chamber pot and washbowl into the slop basin.

Spanner would then bring my breakfast and the *Times* of London to the desk next to the fire. My day had begun. If I were entertaining, Spanner would handle all the details and clean up afterwards. If I was sick in bed, Spanner would bring me my meals. And at night he would place a hot water bottle in my bed before he left.

The water closet I used was a block away, down a ramp, up a ramp. In the rain—it rains all the time in Oxford—the ramps were slippery. The WC itself was a Victorian marble business. The toilet stalls were large enough for my chair, but the doors opened inward, so I had no privacy. The WC was not heated and its windows were kept open all year long, no matter the weather.

The bath facilities were behind the back quadrangle and were inaccessible. I was too shy—or diffident—to ask for help. Accordingly I did not bathe for a year at a time. Neither did I wash my hair. By the end of the year, the buildup of dandruff on my scalp was extraordinary.

The circulation in my legs is poor and I suffered from the cold. My legs would turn blue sometime around October and stay that way until the late spring. I had chilblains that lasted all winter long. I was cold with a dull pain all the time.

Altogether I spent three full years at Oxford. I am exceedingly glad I put up with the hardship, for in spite of all, I learned much, had a wonderful time, and made lifelong friends. I could not stand the hardship now. When I think about it, it is with both awe and pity. No disabled person should have to endure what I willingly went through.

Several years ago, I returned to Oxford for the first time since the 1950s. It was a cold, damp January night; the stone walls were "weeping" on the inside of the buildings as they do in the winter. I started shivering and was very glad when I was back in my warm hotel room in London.

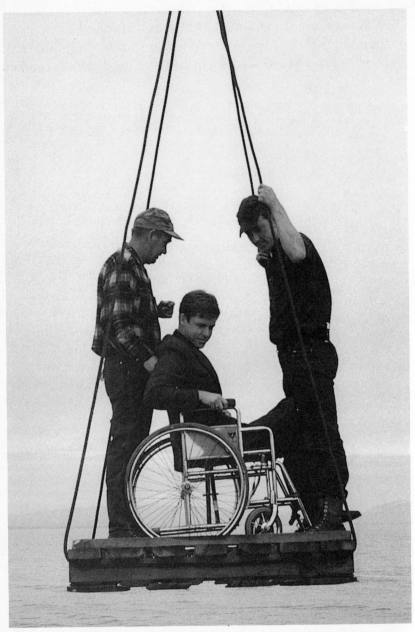

I campaigned in Senator Bartlett's behalf back and forth across the state. Here I am visiting an oil platform in Cook Inlet of the North Pacific Ocean. I am being lifted on a pallet from the deck of the launch used to service the platform. On later platform visits I went by helicopter.

SUCCESS AND BREAKDOWN

I RETURNED TO THE UNITED STATES in the fall of 1959. I had been away three years. I crossed on the old Cunard liner, HMS *Mauritania*. As we steamed into New York harbor, a woman next to me on deck lifted her little girl up so that she could see the Statue of Liberty. There were tears in her eyes.

It was the end of a decade and, as it turned out, the end of an era. For the first half of the century, America had remained a stable society. In spite of two world wars and economic booms and busts, the country had retained its fairly rigid value system. For most Americans, the family was sacrosanct. The man was the breadwinner, the woman the housekeeper. Education of the children was of primary importance. Public institutions were respected—the presidency, the Congress, the press. The government did not lie. America was the greatest land of all.

And indeed it was—and is—but just beneath the surface were much bigotry and injustice. Many people still believed African-Americans were inferior. Many insisted that a woman's place was in the home, that homosexuals were perverts and that the disabled were objects of pity—invalid incompetents who should be kept out of public view.

There was much discrimination in the land of the free and the home of the brave. Most Americans, however, shut their eyes to such problems and went about their business. This was to change in the 1960s and 1970s.

Soon enough, all hell broke loose. There were great conflicts—anger fed by the injustices of prejudice. First came the black revolution and then the women's liberation movement. Students, Native Americans, Hispanics, and gays joined in. All demanded their fair rights and equal opportunities. There was violence, protests, picketing, and marches. From all this the nation emerged as a better society, but the process was not easy and, in the 1990s, it is by no means complete.

The focus of the conflict was Washington, D.C. most especially in the Congress. And I was there. In October of 1959, I went to work for Senator John A. Carroll (D, Colo). At Oxford, I had been the only student using a wheelchair. Again on Capitol Hill, I was the only wheelchair user. Handicap parking did not yet exist. There were steps everywhere; the bathrooms were not accessible but I managed.

With the help of my college friend, soon to be my brother-in-law, Quill Hermans, I moved into an apartment of my own. I had my own hand-controlled car. For the first time, I was on my own—wheelchair and all. My "independent living" life had begun. More than 40 years later, I am still living independently on my own.

Senator Carroll was on the Civil Rights Subcommittee (as it was then named), and I was his staff man for subcommittee business. The civil rights revolution was well underway. The great Senate debates on voting rights, equal accommodations, and public access were underway. They were dramatic and historic and I was there.

For many days and nights, Majority Leader Lyndon Johnson kept the Senate in session around the clock, trying to break the Southern filibuster against legislation mandating equality for African Americans. Tempers rose both in and outside the chamber. Late one night, I had a call from a man who said he would kill me if I did not stop working for equal rights for blacks. I was not the only Senate staffer to get such a call.

In late 1962, I began work for Senator E.L.(Bob) Bartlett (D, Alaska). For the next six years, until his death, I worked closely with Bob on subjects of great import to both of us. I wrote the first anti-Vietnam speech to be given on the Senate floor. Our work on this subject plus my observations of Senators as they debated the Gulf of Tonkin Resolution caused me to ponder the role of foreign policy in the Senate's relationship with the president. In 1964, I obtained a grant from the American Political Science Association, which allowed me to take a year off to write my first book, *Advise and Obstruct: the Senate and Foreign Policy.*[1] The book was a Pulitzer Prize nominee.

While with Bartlett, I initiated studies on Arctic radiation fallout that were used by the Kennedy administration in working out the atmospheric atomic test ban treaty with the Soviet Union. I worked on equal rights for Alaska Natives, which resulted in the Pribilovian Civil Rights Act of 1966. It was at this time I met my lifelong friend, the pioneer Inupiat civil rights leader Charlie Edwardsen. His Inupiat name is Etok. In 1970 I published his biography, *ETOK: A Story of Eskimo Power.*[2] The Alaska Press Club voted it Arctic Book of the Year.

With Bob Bartlett's unfailing support, I began my life's work: the search for equal access and equal rights for disabled people. Over the years, I have written extensively on these issues. I have been responsible for making many of the public buildings of Washington accessible to people with disabilities. I conceived and drafted what became the Federal Architectural Barriers Act of 1968. This is, to my knowledge, the first legislation *anywhere* to treat the equal access of disabled people as a civil right. As such, it was the first step on the road to the Americans with Disabilities Act of 1990.

It was during this period that I also worked a year in the Johnson White House in the old Bureau of the Budget. I wrote what was then called, disrespectfully, "Rose Garden Garbage." These were signing statements, veto messages, etc. Some were important, most were trivial. All were most carefully written and coordinated with the various interested federal departments and agencies. I learned there is no room for creativity, let alone humor, in papers of state.

---

[1]Delacorte Press, New York, NY, 1965
[2]Putnams & Sons, New York, NY, 1970

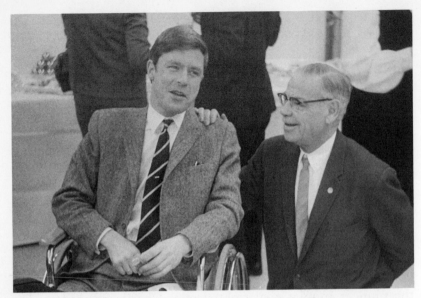

Here I am with my boss, Senator E.L.(Bob) Bartlett (D, Alaska). Bob was a great man, "the Father of Alaska Statehood." The occasion was a party held for campaign workers after the Senator's 80% re-election victory.

During these years I was busy and I was productive. My life was devoted to my work. I had no private life. My paralyzed body was my obedient servant: it did what I forced it to do. I was numb to its aches and pains. I received no pleasure from it, sexual or otherwise. Today it is a popular cliche to "listen" to one's body, to pay attention to one's feelings. I knew nothing of this. As I was to learn later, this is a foolish way to live—and dangerous.

The 1970s were good years for the disability rights movement. The Architectural Barriers Act was amended to include public transportation. Added later was the Architectural and Transportation Barriers Compliance Board with powers to enforce the terms of the act. The concept of the Architectural Barriers Act was broadly extended by Section 504 in the Rehabilitation Act of 1973. This section reads, "No otherwise qualified individual in the United States shall, solely by reason of his handicap be excluded from participation in, be denied the benefits of, or be subject to discrimination under any program or activity receiving Federal assistance."

The Ford and Carter administrations were reluctant to issue the regulations necessary for the enforcement of Section 504. Disability activists, including such leaders as Judy Heumann, Ed Roberts, and Mary Jane Owen, seized and occupied the offices of the Department of Health and Human Services across the country. This action generated an immense amount of publicity and attention; only then did the Carter administration finally promulgate the regulations, April 28, 1977.

Perhaps the most important disability rights act of all, the Education Act of 1974, mandated the "mainstreaming" of disabled children whenever possible into public school classrooms. Over the years this has served two purposes. It has produced a generation of young persons with disabilities who have learned how to live independently in the world of the able-bodied. It has also demonstrated to able-bodied children that the disabled are not objects of fear and strangeness, but rather, ordinary people like themselves. This has helped enormously to reduce discrimination based on ignorance.

Major disability rights legislation was approved in the 1970s. Curiously, this legislation was largely conceived and steered through the Congress *in behalf* of disabled people, not *by* disabled people themselves. In fact, a large part of the disability rights agenda was passed into law before the disability rights movement had formed or learned how to exert its power. The success of the civil rights movement and women's liberation efforts made the public and the politicians sensitive to injustices wherever present in our society. Women and African Americans had demanded and received guarantees that their rights would be protected. So when the question was asked, "Why shouldn't the disabled have the same guarantees," the answer was clear: Simple justice required that disabled people should have access to the polling booth, education, jobs, transportation, et al.

The disabled were an oppressed minority. Furthermore, they were a large minority. Every American, who is not himself disabled, has a family member or a friend who is. Disability cuts across political lines; both liberals and conservatives know disability. There is political sex appeal in disability issues.

At first, Senators and Congressmen thought that disability rights was a free vote. It was what is called a "motherhood" issue—a vote that cost no money and angered no group. Congress had for years been approving an annual "Hire the Handicapped Week" resolution.

At first, the Congress saw disability rights as no more important or costly. By the end of the decade, they had learned differently. Disability rights would not be free.

First in Berkeley, California—with the independent living movement and the Disability Rights, Education and Defense Fund—and then spreading across the country, disabled people began to organize. Parents of disabled children began to organize. All these people, and they were many, were determined that what had been promised, in fact, would be delivered. This would take both motivation and money.

My focus in the 1970s was not upon this movement; it was, alas, upon myself.

After the death of Senator Bartlett at the end of 1968, I went to work for British Petroleum, Ltd., one of the five largest companies in the world. BP had never had a significant operation in the United States, but with the discovery of oil on its Alaska holdings, BP became at one strike the company with the largest crude reserves in America. I was its chief political officer and it was my job to explain the complexities of our congressional, federal form of government to a puzzled board of directors in the London home office. I was with the company for five years. These were busy and heady years. In the world of Washington politics and lobbying, I was playing with the "Big Boys."

While my professional career was going well, all was not well with my private life. In fact, I had no private life. All my energy and effort were invested in maintaining the shaky facade I presented to the world. There was nothing behind it.

Finally, on the 4th of July weekend, 1974, my body and soul rebelled. I went home from my office and never went back. I had collapsed both mentally and physically. I found myself in the grip of a deep situational depression, and I spent the rest of the decade getting out of it.

The following section contains pieces I wrote—during and about—these two eventful decades.

EARLY DAYS IN DISABILITY RIGHTS

I have written this piece especially for this book. Never before have I written about these early projects of the disability movement. Since their inception, they have developed over the years into major nation-wide, even worldwide efforts. I hope you will find their beginnings of interest. Today it is hard to believe that only 25 years ago, official Washington was inaccessible to disabled citizens.

IT IS NOT OFTEN that one is in a position to effect real change. I was in such a position from 1963 through 1968. During these years, I was employed by the senior Senator from Alaska, Bob Bartlett. The Senator authorized me to work on disability issues. He agreed to support me in this work, just as long as it did not interfere with my other responsibilities.

In these years, with Senator Bartlett behind me, I was able to help make Washington's public buildings and monuments accessible for disabled people; to improve accessibility at the nation's parks, hospitals and airports; and to establish a disability rights precedent which, a generation later, continues to grow and flourish.

To accomplish these things, I piggy-backed on the power and good will that my boss, Senator Bob Bartlett of Alaska, had built up during his twenty year career in the Congress. Bob was a member of the Senate "inner circle," well-known and well-liked in official Washington. He was a member of the Commerce and the Appropriations Committees.

As his Legislative (later Administrative) Assistant, I worked closely with him, and a strong mutual trust developed between us. So strong in fact, that during his last year when he was often in hospital with heart disease, I acted in his behalf, recording his votes. ("If present and voting, the Senator from Alaska would vote aye.") I also issued policy statements in his name and made committee decisions for him. I briefed him on my actions only as his health condition allowed. He never repudiated my decisions—thank God!

My first disability project concerned the Library of Congress. The Library is by law a creature of the Congress. It is not a part of the executive branch of our federal government. In addition to being the largest library in the world and the American depository of record, it is also a service agency for the Congress. The costs of its operations are provided for in the Legislative Appropriations Bill. Senator Bartlett happened to be Chairman of the Subcommittee responsible for this measure.

As part of my duties with the Senator, I had cause to go to the Library from time to time to research an issue or find background for a speech. The Library was not accessible. The front door was an old, heavy, revolving affair, with five short, high steps leading to it. This would be tough to ramp. The back doors, however, would be easy to make accessible. There was one shallow step up to a platform, and but one more step from the platform to the door.

I drafted a letter to the Librarian of Congress, Quincy Mumford, and Bartlett signed it. The letter asked that a simple ramp be built at one of the back entrances. The matter quickly became a federal case. The Library was not anxious to irritate Chairman Bartlett. On the other hand, it was a conservative institution under Mumford, and change was not something to be rushed without considerable deliberation. There had never been a ramp at the door. Was it a good policy, was it, perhaps, wise, at this late date, to put one there now? A committee was appointed, deliberations held, and, finally, at last, a letter emerged in response to the Senator's inquiry. A ramp could be built, but the Architect of the Capitol would have to be consulted. The authority of the Librarian to make a physical addition to the physical plant of the Library, without the direct expression of the Congress, must be investigated. Perhaps the Joint Congressional Committee of the Library would need to be consulted, and, in addition, there was no money available for the ramp.

The Senator was a man who contained his emotions well. He was extremely quick-witted, highly intelligent, easily bored, and often terribly tired, a man with little patience. All of this was largely and usually hidden behind a genial facade like an old shoe. This impenetrable geniality made his departures from it all the more memorable. The Senator called the Librarian to his office and lost his temper. He had asked for a ramp, and they had given him gobbledygook. The Librarian replied that, be that as it may, a ramp would cost $5,000 and would require a specific act of Congress. The Senator said, so be it. And that is why there was a line item, a specific direction in the Legislative Appropriations Act of 1964 that allocated $5,000 for the construction of a ramp at the Library of Congress.

The Library, for reasons unknown, chose to build its ramp of sheet iron. It is the only sheet iron ramp I have ever seen, but it is still there, as strong as the day it was built. The Library invited me to lunch the day it was completed, and we had a small, informal dedication ceremony, as I rolled my wheelchair unassisted up and down the ramp, in and out of the Library.

Several months later, I happened to ask a member of the custodial staff if many other wheelchair users had used the ramp. "No," he said thoughtfully, "although we have had several people sprain their ankles on it." I suggested that we just keep that information between ourselves.

Since then the new Librarian, James Billington, has worked with real dedication to turn the Library into a model of accessibility. The Library has dramatically improved its facilities. Special parking places are designated; rest rooms have been altered; study aids, such as lapboards, are available. The front entrance has been completely redesigned: the steps are gone as is the revolving door. The driveway has been elevated, providing a level entrance, and the doors are electrically opened, activated by pressure plates on the floor. The Library has come far in 15 years—both in its facilities for, and in its sensitivity to, the handicapped. Bartlett's display of temper has paid off for the benefit of many crippled scholars and tourists—and at least one Senate staff aide.

The National Gallery of Art plays an important part in my life. I obtain enormous pleasure from my visits. It is a blessing to have access to this world-class collection of paintings and sculpture. "*Access*" is the key word in that sentence. When I worked for Senator Bartlett, the Gallery was not accessible. The Mall side entrance has many, many steps but the Constitution Avenue entrance is practically level. It has but two shallow steps. It seemed to me that a small wooden ramp, not more than 10 inches high, would make it possible for me to visit the Gallery without assistance. I would be able to visit the collections when I wanted, look at the pictures as long as I wanted without being dependent upon the help or acquiescence of others. Bartlett required us to work Saturday mornings and there was many a Saturday afternoon that I would have stopped at the Gallery on my way home, if there had been a ramp.

The Senator was a member of the Appropriations Subcommittee that funds the Smithsonian Museums and the National Gallery of Art. Accordingly, using Appropriations Committee stationery, I wrote a letter for Bartlett's signature to the Director of the Gallery, John Walker, asking that a modest ramp be built so that disabled tourists and visitors would have access to the Gallery on the same basis as the able-bodied.

Walker said no. He replied that a ramp was not necessary. There was always a guard stationed at the entrance, and he was instructed to provide any assistance necessary to help disabled people enter the building. This answer was not what I was after. I like to be independent, I don't like asking strangers for assistance and, besides, I thought I had a right to enter this public building just as easily as any other taxpayer. Accordingly, I developed a plan. I would use myself as a test case to prove to Walker that the present system did not work. I had observed that, although on fair days the guards were at the door ready to help, on inclement days they stayed inside behind the security desk, out of sight of disabled people needing help.

So on a snowy Saturday afternoon, I went alone to the Gallery, watch in hand, to see just how long it took for a guard to notice and assist me into the building. It was cold and miserable but I was determined to prove my point. The driveway was empty, there was even a parking place close to the door. I got my chair out of the car and sloshed through the wet snow to the bottom of the steps. Just then, out of nowhere, appeared two French tourists. Before I knew it, they were pulling my chair up the steps. "No," I was saying, "No, you don't understand. I am waiting for a guard to come out and help me." Too late! Already, I was up the steps and into the building.

So, at least that time, Walker was right about getting into the building. I, however, was right about the principle of the thing and I was not about to give up. In a further exchange of letters, Director Walker again said no, he was sorry, but a ramp would do harm to the architectural integrity of the building. This seemed silly to me: a 10 inch ramp could not do *much* harm. But the Director had made up his mind. He concluded his reply by writing that, if Bartlett wished to pursue the matter further, he would have to take it up with the Board of Trustees whose Chairman was the Chief Justice of the United States Supreme Court, Earl Warren.

I drafted a letter for the Senator's signature to each of the members of the Board asking that a ramp be built. The ramp matter was placed on the agenda of the Board's annual meeting. The day before the meeting, Bartlett called the Chief Justice who promised he would do what he could. Warren, whose daughter "Honeybear" had polio not many years before, called Bartlett after the meeting, "Bob, we've got our ramp!" According to the Chief Justice, the board had approved unanimously the construction of a ramp at the Gallery entrance.

Walker, who knew a *fait accompli* when he saw one, changed sides. He wrote the Senator, "I am delighted to say that the Trustees voted unanimously for a ramp . . . which will allow anyone in a wheelchair to enter the Gallery without the problem of the two steps. . . . With appreciation of your interest in the National Gallery and your helpfulness in this matter, etc, etc."

A "temporary," 10 inch high wooden ramp—costing no more than a hundred dollars—was built at once. I went to try it out. As I reported in a letter from Bartlett to Director Walker, "My friend in a wheelchair of whom I have spoken in the past tells me that he visited the Gallery Saturday afternoon. He made the visit alone. He tells me he was very much impressed by the temporary ramp in place. It is satisfactory in every way and he is delighted with it. Of course he tells me he was even more delighted with your new Rembrandt."

Although Walker said that planning was underway for the construction of a permanent ramp, it was more than 25 years before the "temporary" was replaced by a tasteful granite ramp. The architectural integrity of the National Gallery remains intact.

Recently, I learned that Walker as a child had contracted polio. This left him ambulatory but weak. I am told he kept himself as thin as possible to minimize the burden his muscles had to carry. Even so, his weakened muscles caused him much fatigue and pain. Nevertheless, he refused to favor or otherwise accommodate his disability, handling it with discipline and denial. This attitude toward his own condition was perhaps a factor in his opposition to the ramp.

Edmund Leonard was a young man who worked for what was then called the President's Committee for the Employment of the Handicapped. This was—and is—largely a symbolic operation. This committee has personnel but no clear authority or responsibility. Although the agency did not do much, Ed did. He was enthusiastic and motivated. Over the years, we cooked up several excellent things.

One day at lunch, Ed Leonard and I came up with an idea for a guide for handicapped visitors to the National Parks. Senator Bartlett was a member of the Interior Appropriations Subcommittee. Although the aged Senator Hayden was Chairman of the Subcommittee, it was Bartlett who usually acted as Chairman at the meetings of the Subcommittee. In other words, the National Park Service knew that the Senator had a large say in determining the size of their annual budget. The Park Service was anxious to be of service.

Senator Bartlett wrote the Service, asking that a survey be made of each park and monument as to accessibility: steps, trails, toilet facilities. Bartlett said that the information, once obtained, would be compiled and organized by the handicapped themselves at no expense to the government. Ed Leonard, working with the Crippled Children Association and others, had volunteered to find the needed editors.

The Park Service agreed to the survey, and, soon, the material began flooding into the office. There are a great many parks and monuments, but Leonard was as good as his word. The material was edited and organized, and the Parks Service printed it with a foreword written by the Senator, congratulating all concerned. This was in 1965. The Easter Seal Society had assembled guides for the handicapped to some of the larger cities of varying reliability and usefulness, but this was the first guide published by the federal government and the first comprehensive guide for the use of the handicapped published anywhere. Over time, the parks' guide was expanded and greater detail added. A new edition was issued every year. It was kept in print for many years, and hundreds of thousands of copies were distributed. The guide is now privately printed.

I believe the guide gave the Park Service an early awareness of the needs of its disabled visitors. The various parks and monuments began to compete informally to make their facilities more accessible. As a result, the National Park Service has pioneered in the development of nature trails for the blind, mountain access for people using wheelchairs, and other innovative ways of bringing the wilderness experience to the handicapped.

Later, Ed Leonard called me to say that the 3M Company had sent him some Scotch Lite signs of a little stick person using a wheelchair. He thought they might be useful for store owners to indicate accessibility. He brought them over to my office, and I thought they were nifty.

It seemed to me that we should really encourage their widespread use. Ed thought that if we were going to do that, how could we be sure they would not be misused? An unscrupulous merchant might put one on a bathroom door when the bathroom was not really accessible. He was right. I could well imagine a wheelchair user getting stuck in the john. Ed asked, "shouldn't Congress pass a law of some sort, setting standards for its use?"

After some thought, I disagreed. Rather than placing restrictions on its use, shouldn't we do all we could to support its use across the country? This would serve two purposes: it would signal to the disabled where they were welcome and, at the same time, it would increase the able-bodied public awareness of disabled people and the problems they have with accessibility. The sign had symbolic as well as practical value.

Ed came around to my thinking. Now the sign is in universal, worldwide use. But Ed Leonard was right about the dangers of its misuse. I am sure I am not the only wheelchair user who has been trapped in an inaccessible bathroom with an accessible sign on its door!

The General Services Administration was anxious to demonstrate to Senator Bartlett its concern for the handicapped. Accordingly, it put out a press release stating that the new federal office building at Juneau, the state capitol of Alaska, was to be the first in the nation to be constructed with complete accessibility for the handicapped. The Senator was asked to inspect the new building, and, as he was unable to do so, I was asked to take his place.

Our car was met at the door by the building's administrator, the builder, and the regional GSA director. I got out of the car with my wheelchair, shook hands all around, and said, "Let's go." The inspection, as it turned out, was a tour from top to bottom of the just-finished building. GSA really had made an effort. There was one reserved parking place near the front door. The door itself was level. The elevator buttons were in reach of a person in a wheelchair. One of the men's rooms had an accessible toilet stall as did one of the women's rooms in the eight-story building. I asked to see the accessible male rest room. "Right you are," said the GSA director. "Say, what floor is it on, Charlie," he asked the builder.

"Well," the builder hesitated, "I guess it's on four."

So, we went up to four. But it was not on four. We tried five. It was not on five. By now, there was a certain tension in the proceedings. We started on the bottom floor and looked at every men's room on every floor, floor after floor. Not one was accessible. By now, feelings were running high, and there were grumbled recriminations, not entirely out of my earshot, between the builder and the GSA executive. In desperation, we began looking in the ladies' rooms. We inspected every single ladies' room, and not one of them was accessible.

As finally pieced together, the explanation was that the specification for one accessible bathroom for each sex was, indeed, in the original contract; but transmission of the directions between contractor and subcontractor had somehow mysteriously failed. No one, either with the builder's firm or with GSA, had thought to make an inspection at the time of the building's completion and transfer.

This illustrates nicely the challenge facing the handicapped. Vigilance is more than the price of liberty; it is the cost of an accessible bathroom. All the laws on the books can be as strong as possible, but unless handicapped citizens demand the enforcement of the law, insist upon the equal exercise of their equal rights to access to any and all buildings and programs supported by tax funds, and unless the handicapped are vigilant and persistent, society will forget.

1997 was the 25th anniversary of the Kennedy Center here in Washington. To mark the occasion, the building underwent a $50 million renovation. According to the Center's President, Lawrence J. Wilker, the renovation was necessary to bring it up to the standards of the Americans with Disabilities Act. He said, "As the nation's center for the performing arts, we have the responsibility to be in the forefront of accessibility."

My! Thinking at the Center has come a long way in 25 years. The John F. Kennedy Center for the Performing Arts, as originally designed by Edward Durrell Stone, was inaccessible to mobility-impaired people.

In the mid 1950s, it was proposed to construct a national cultural center on the banks of the Potomac. This was to be built and operated on a privately-funded basis. Plans were drawn, committees organized and money raised. First Lady Mamie Eisenhower lent her name as honorary chairman. By 1963, the drive had lost its momentum and the project languished.

It was President Johnson's idea to resuscitate the cultural center project by naming it as the national memorial to his predecessor, the assassinated President, John Kennedy. Accordingly, Johnson asked the Congress to appropriate Federal funds to finance construction of the building. Senator Bartlett was Acting Chairman of the Interior Appropriations Subcommittee that had Senate jurisdiction over this proposal.

The proposal was controversial. The Congress was anxious to honor Kennedy, but extremely reluctant to get into show business as a theater owner. Contrary to popular belief, the Congress does care about the expenditure of the public's tax money, and the Kennedy Center was a venture into an area without federal precedent. After a good deal of discussion, a compromise was agreed upon: the building would be constructed with federal funds and maintained as a national monument by the National Park Service, but the productions—the plays, operas, and concerts—would be privately funded and managed.

Bartlett was a popular man in the Congress. If Bartlett approved the project, so would his committee, the Senate, and the Congress. If he did not approve, it would be difficult, if not impossible, to obtain the funds. In the face of his opposition the Kennedy Center would not be built. And the Johnson administration knew this.

I talked with the Senator. We agreed this situation presented us with an opportunity to insist that accessibility for the disabled be incorporated into the overall architectural design of the building. We believed that the Center should be accessible to all Americans as a matter of right. We thought it should be accessible as a tribute to the late President's interest in the disabled, both mental and physical. And we thought it should be accessible as a model to the nation of what a public building could be.

The building, as originally designed, had steps leading from the grand foyer into the opera house, the theatre, and the concert hall. There were no access ramps to these halls. There was no level access from the basement garage to the elevators. There was no reserved handicap parking in these garages and no curb cuts anywhere. The bathrooms were inaccessible.

February 25, 1964, writing under Bartlett's signature, I addressed these issues in letters to architect Stone and the Director of the Kennedy Center project, Roger Stevens. The letter spoke of the Kennedy family's interest in disabled persons and their problems. Bartlett said that the concept of the cultural center as the national memorial to the late president had his support and added that he was sure Stone and Stevens would agree that its cultural facilities should be "fully accessible" to the disabled. He added that the Royal Festival

Hall and the new Lincoln Center were accessible and stated, "I know you will agree that the Kennedy Center should be as well." We received no reply to my letter. After several months, I wrote again. Again, we received no reply. When Stevens and Stone came before the Senator's Subcommittee considering the Center's request for construction funds, Bartlett asked in person what we had asked by letter. The response was less than satisfying. In fact, *no* consideration had been given to the needs of the disabled. There would be steps into each of the three theatres. Bathrooms would be standard; toilet stalls unaccessible. There would be no parking provisions.

And, so, after the hearing, I called Stevens. I told him the Senator and his subcommittee would take no action whatsoever on the Kennedy Center appropriation request. No action, that is, until the Senator was assured the Center would to be accessible to all Americans.

When the officials of the Center determined that the Senator was serious and that he had the votes necessary to block the project, there was a sudden and permanent reverse in policy. Plans were redrawn, experts were consulted, and the Center became a model of convenience and accessibility for the handicapped. The handicapped were made to feel welcome. As a result, the number of disabled people attending the Center has grown each year, and the Center is rightly proud of its role as a leader and model in this area. Theatres and cultural centers across the country have benefitted from the Kennedy Center's example.

Senator Bartlett and I blackmailed Stevens and Stone, but it was for their own good.

Lister Hill was a distinguished Senator from Alabama. He was the coauthor of the Hill-Burton hospital construction program. This program made it possible for communities in every state in the country to construct modern, state-of-the-art health facilities in the years after World War II. These facilities were being built without thought to the accessibility needs of disabled people. It is one of the ironies of the times that hospitals were so inaccessible. Private bathrooms and the stalls of public bathrooms were too small; beds were too high; entrances had steps.

When the bill reauthorizing the Hill-Burton program came to the floor, I had ready an amendment directing that hospitals built with federal funds should be made accessible for disabled people. Bartlett talked to his friend, Lister Hill. Hill agreed to accept the amendment and it was done. Just like that. Today, close to 30 years later, virtually every hospital in the land is accessible to disabled people.

After our successful intervention at the National Gallery, I turned my attention to the museums of the Smithsonian Institution. These great buildings lining the Mall, from the Capitol to the Washington Monument, are the most popular museums in the world. Then and now, millions of tourists a year pass through the doors of these museums. Back in the 1960s however, these museums were virtually inaccessible to the handicapped. I made repeated appeals (in Bartlett's name) to S. Dillon Ripley, Secretary of the Smithsonian. We received several detailed reports on accessibility, which gave the appearance of interest and concern with the problem, but which were, in fact, deceptive and misleading. For example, Mr. Ripley said there was no problem entering the Freer Gallery of Art because there was a level entrance on Constitution Avenue. There was, indeed, such an entrance, but it was kept locked from inside and could only be unlocked—with obvious reluctance—by appeal to the guards at the main entrance seated at a desk located at the head of a formidable flight of stairs. It was a paradoxical situation. The independent handicapped person could only avoid the stairs by climbing the stairs.

Stairs were everywhere. Fountains, phones, and bathrooms were inaccessible. Not only were the toilet stall doors too narrow, but the very corridors into the bathrooms of the Arts and Sciences building were too narrow to allow a wheelchair to pass. Bartlett brought up such matters in appropriations hearings, but the Smithsonian Institution is a venerable and largely independent operation with a private endowment and appropriated funds. Its policies are set by the Secretary and its Board of Regents, and the Board of Regents would not be swayed by Bartlett's arguments. The Board was convinced there was no problem, and admitting no problem, they did nothing to rectify it.

We had struck out. There was nothing we could do to make the Smithsonian accessible—short of an act of Congress. This got me to thinking: What about an act of Congress?

Drafting legislation is an extremely specialized skill. Unless a law is carefully and specifically crafted it may not have the effect intended and it may indeed have completely unintended consequences. One day in 1966, I went down to the Legislative Counsel and met with Blair Crownover. I asked him to help me draft a bill that would require that all buildings, built wholly or in part with federal tax funds, should be designed to be accessible to all citizens. Such an approach was used in the 1960s civil rights legislation I worked on with both Senators Carroll and Bartlett. I have always seen the equal access of disabled people to buildings, transportation, employment and, indeed, to society, as a civil rights issue. Disabled Americans should have all the rights granted to other citizens. They are taxpayers just like anyone else and they should have the same access to programs and facilities funded by their tax dollars as do able-bodied persons.

I wanted the bill to be framed in civil rights language. I wanted it to be simple. I wanted accessibility to be one of the items on the checklist that federal contractors must comply with: fire standards, electric safety standards and, according to my thought, accessibility. Finally, I asked that the bill be drafted so that, upon its introduction, the Parliamentarian would refer it to the Public Works Committee. This was the committee with jurisdiction over Federal buildings and facilities. I particularly did not want it referred to what was then called the Labor and Public Welfare Committee. This was where all previous "disability" legislation had gone. In those days, disabled people were seen, by and large, in a medical context. They were sick people who never got well.

The Labor and Public Welfare Committee, although chaired by the distinguished Alabama Senator Lister Hill, was completely controlled, so far as disabled people were concerned, by Mary Switzer, the lifetime head of Vocational Rehabilitation. Miss Switzer was a consummate bureaucrat and lobbyist. She was also an empire-builder. She wanted anything having anything to do with people with disabilities in her agency. She was an able person, and no doubt, did much good but I saw her as patronizing to disabled people. She saw them as her flock, perhaps her children. She did not like me nor—as the reader might guess—did I care all that much for her.

If the bill had gone to Hill's Committee, it undoubtedly would have emerged, if it emerged at all, with the Department of Health, Education and Welfare in charge, drafting regulations and building standards for U.S. public buildings. HEW (now HHS) was—and is—highly bureaucratic. They would have made a fine mess of the business.

When I took the draft bill to Bartlett, he agreed to introduce it for Senate consideration. This involved dropping the bill in "the hopper," a box on the Senate Parliamentarian's desk. The Parliamentarian then looks it over and decides which committee to refer the proposed legislation. I was at his desk as he read Bartlett's bill. He decided to refer it to Hill's Labor and Public Welfare Committee—certain death, I felt.

"Oh no," I pleaded. "It's not about the handicapped. It's about buildings, about architecture and standards."

"Well, in that case," the Parliamentarian responded after some thought, "I shall refer it to the Public Works Committee which has responsibility for public buildings."

I was greatly relieved.

Now it was necessary to find a sponsor in the House of Representatives to introduce the bill in the House. This was easy. Charles Bennett was a Congressman from Florida. He had polio and wore long leg braces. Furthermore, he was an old friend of the Senator. Bartlett called him and asked him to sponsor the bill. Bennett was pleased to give his support. In fact, upon his retirement some 25 years later, he cited the Architectural Barriers Act as the proudest achievement of his Congressional career.

When Miss Switzer learned that Senator Bartlett was planning to introduce a bill on architectural barriers, she went to the Health and Public Welfare Committee and got them to add an amendment to an authorization bill creating a presidential commission to study the issue and report on what Federal policy should be. Senator Bartlett and I did not learn of the Commission until it had become law.

Switzer's ploy was a classic Washington strategy: If a decision is about to be made that you oppose, do anything you can to delay the decision. Nothing delays a decision better than a commission; it can study the issue, and study, and study.

Miss Switzer would serve as *rapporteur* and draft its final report. It is not surprising that the final report recommended that architectural barriers become one of the responsibilities of Vocational Rehabilitation, Mary Switzer's agency.

Fortunately, the Chairman of the Senate Public Works Committee, Jennings Randolph, the senior Senator of West Virginia, was a good friend of Bartlett's. Randolph was a Senator of the old school. He was portly with a florid face. Whenever he passed me in the hall, he would greet me with, "How are you, dear heart?" and pat me on the shoulder. He was a softie for disabled people.

As a member of the Appropriations Committee, Bob Bartlett had done many a favor for Randolph and his needy state of West Virginia. Randolph was pleased to return a favor for good old Bob. He gave the bill his very powerful support.

Copies of the bill were sent by the Committee to the federal agencies that would be affected if the bill became law. The agencies were asked to comment on the proposal and its possible effects. In those days, the agencies sent their comments for clearance to the Bureau of the Budget (now OMB). The Bureau's responsibility was to see that the agencies' views were consistent and coordinated with the policies of the President. The Bureau would then prepare its own cover report, stating whether the Administration supported, had no objection, or opposed passage of the legislation.

In the case of the Architectural Barriers Act, the Johnson administration opposed passage. This was at the height of the Vietnam War as well as the War on Poverty. LBJ's "guns and butter" budgets were wildly out of control. The Bureau of the Budget was afraid that the Bartlett legislation would cost money—as indeed over the years, it has. Furthermore, the Bureau added in its report that such legislation was not needed. President Eisenhower had once issued a proclamation calling upon federal agencies to make appropriate arrangements for handicapped citizens, and the Bureau was sure that everything that could be done was being done. In any case, it was prudent to await the report of the Architectural Barriers Commission.

The opposition of the administration was a serious setback. Senator Bartlett was not a "showboat" senator. He did not introduce legislation simply for press attention. If he introduced a bill, he did so because he meant for it to become law. We pressed ahead. Chairman Randolph scheduled hearings. By that time, close to 20 Senators had co-sponsored the Bartlett bill. Many of them had submitted statements in support.

The summer and fall of 1968, I was in Alaska acting in the Senator's behalf as state coordinator of the much-benighted Hubert Humphrey campaign for president. Back in Washington, Jack Cornman, our press man, worked on behalf of the Architectural Barriers bill. It was he who worked with the House and Senate Committees. The Pentagon was adamantly against the bill, and it was Jack who negotiated a compromise that exempted the armed forces from coverage. Without this exemption, the bill never would have passed.

It was an election year, the nation was torn asunder by antiwar protests, assassinations, and the hippie revolution. The politicians on Capitol Hill were worried about reelection. Something as good-sounding, cheap (or so they thought), and noncontroversial as helping the handicapped appeared to them to be a real vote winner. When the Committee reported the bill favorably to the whole Senate, it was therefore brought up promptly on the floor and passed without objection.

When the bill was called up for consideration on the House side, it passed so quickly without objection that members were unable to register their support for it. Accordingly, a roll call vote was called so that each member could record his "Aye," in support of accessibility for the handicapped.

I always thought President Johnson displayed more than usual *chutzpah* when he staged a full-scale signing ceremony to sign the bill into law. After all, this was the bill his administration had opposed.

★ ★ ★ ★

I had been talking with Senator Robert Kennedy's office in the spring of 1968. We were planning to introduce legislation in the next Congress to amend the Minimum Wage Act to include disabled people working in the so-called sheltered workshops. These people worked full time, worked as hard as they could, and yet were still dependent on their families because of the miserably low wages they were paid. We were going to argue: an honest day's pay for an honest day's work. If the sheltered workshop could not afford this, then we proposed a government subsidy to cover the gap.

Alas, Bobby Kennedy was shot and killed in the summer and Bob Bartlett died in the fall. I left Capitol Hill, my Cinderella days over. I lost my power and became just another working stiff. But, with Bartlett's help, much had been accomplished, much that I am proud of.

A Visit to
Flat, Alaska

For over ten years I went to Alaska at least once or twice a year. When I worked for Senator Bartlett, I would stay three or four months at a time. The naturalist John Muir once said that the traveler should save Alaska for last. Alaska has such spectacular beauty that it makes everywhere else look like small potatoes. I grew to love Alaska's beauty and all the friends I made in the state.

I was the Alaska state coordinator for the 1964 Lyndon Johnson presidential campaign and in 1968 for the Humphrey campaign. In 1966, I managed Bob Bartlett's Senate campaign and arranged a presidential visit. As Bartlett's representative, I traveled all over the state from Nome to Fort Yukon, Ketchikan to Barrow.

I traveled by dogsled, helicopter, and speedboat. I was carried "fireman's carry," up and down the ladders of a gold dredge; I was lifted by crane from a little boat in the middle of Cook Inlet up onto an oil platform. I stayed in a miner's cabin, an Eskimo home, a Quonset-hut hotel with the cubicles separated from each other by sheets hanging on clothes lines and a "honey bucket" at the end of the hall. I saw many whales, hundreds of bears, thousands of caribou. I saw the northern *lights and volcanoes erupting. I was in an earthquake that measured more than seven on the Richter Scale. I was stranded in my car, 30 miles from anywhere, at 10 degrees below zero. I crash-landed my AeroCoupe airplane. I drove into a moose. I had a hell of a time.*

Here is an example. This is a report I wrote to Senator Bartlett after a visit to Flat.

OCTOBER 1964

On Saturday and Sunday, October 10 and 11, 1964, I visited Flat, Alaska. Flat is an old and largely deserted mining town, approximately 350 miles northwest of Anchorage. There is no road to Flat; there never has been. Located on one of the tributaries of the Yukon River, the town was originally settled by miners who walked in from Fairbanks. Supplies and equipment were barged up the Yukon. Now, of course, the only way in or out is by plane.

I flew up with Hugh Matheson, Bobby Sholton, and Maury Carlson. The three were roommates in Anchorage before their marriages. They are old and good friends, and every fall they try to get up to Flat, at least for a weekend, to see and talk with their old mining buddies and perhaps to shoot a moose. Hunting is by far the least important part of their trip. I was extremely pleased they asked me to go along. I had a wonderful and extraordinary time.

Hugh, of course, is an old gold-miner himself. He mined for years up in the Chandalar in the Brooks Range. Hugh loves the life and would very much like to go back to it, if only he could find a stream with enough certain pay to insure that he could get his kids through school on the proceeds. Such streams are hard to come by. Bobby and Maury are both ex-bush pilots. They have flown everything everywhere in Alaska. They are, of course, the guys who own the two famous flying boxcars, which have taken up so much of the FAA's time as of late. They are good pilots and mechanics. They keep their planes in good shape, but they just do not understand, and rebel at, bureaucratic or unwilling regulations. You will remember, a few months back, that the FAA in a formal report to Senator Bartlett

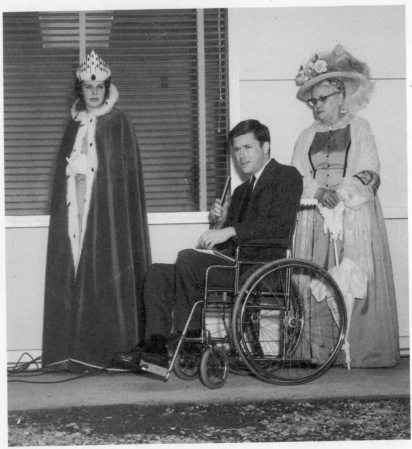

My first speech in Alaska, June 22, 1963. I was dedicating an air flight service station at the Nome Festival of the Midnight Sun. That is Midnight Sun Queen Ann Chambers on the left and Mrs. Chrissy Waldhelm on the right. Chrissy was the oldest surviving pioneer of the Nome gold rush of 1901. She spent the first bitterly cold winter living in a tent on the shore of the Bering Sea. She told me that what she remembered of the experience: "It was just party, party, party from tent to tent."

complained that Maury had used abusive and profane language in talking to one of the FAA inspectors. When I asked Maury about this, he said, "Hell, I should have hit him with a two-by-four."

Sholton and Carlson have a surplus two-engine Beachcraft, which we used to fly into Flat. The day of the flight was a beautiful clear sunny day, the first we have had in over a month. They insisted that I sit in the copilot's seat, and I was, of course, delighted to do so. The flight was superb. Bobby flew low over the mountains, and we crossed the Alaska range, went north along it to Rainy Pass, only 30 or 40 miles southwest of Mt. McKinley. All the mountains were snow-covered, pure white, rough, and jagged. Mts. McKinley and Foraker were huge, rising masses on the horizon. We went through Rainy Pass below the level of the peaks on either side, and it was exciting in the way that a roller coaster is exciting. Contributing to the excitement was the fact that something began to smoke in the cockpit, just as we were going through the pass. We could see the smoke, we could smell it, but we could not find its source. This caused a good deal of interest. We sniffed and sniffed and sniffed all over the cabin. We never did find the source, and as Bobby said, "You can't expect everything to go good." This, of course, was not as reassuring as it might have been, or rather, as one might have liked. Nothing, however, actually stopped going. For the rest of the flight, Bobby and I kept telling each other that the smell was going away—although neither of us believed it to be true.

During the course of the flight, I flew a bit myself. I did not mind too much taking the controls over the Yukon Valley, but taking them when the plane was over the mountains was rather unnerving. The thing about flying a plane is that you can go any which way, not only left and right, but up and down, as well. Unlike driving on a road, you cannot see the bumps before you hit them. Bobby and Maury operate their airplanes the same way that my Uncle Tim operates his cars—the engines are always in excellent condition, but the door handles and trunk knobs keep falling off. While we were at Flat, Maury lost a piece of the airplane that he had in his pocket, and we all had to spend an hour or so looking for it—in the pickup, on the floor of the cabin, etc.

As we came into Flat, we circled around the mountain outside town and buzzed the Agoff and the Fullerton mining camps before landing in downtown Flat. We just beat the fog in. There was a black bear on the hill, watching us as we came in.

We were met at the plane by Johnny Miscovich, who drove us down in his pickup to his house for a drink and to meet his wife, Mary. Johnny's family has been at Flat for 30 years. He is renting a dredge on Otter Creek. It is one of the last two or three dredges still operating in Alaska. Johnny is the Republican candidate for the State Legislature, and I cannot help hoping that he wins. Rich Fullerton drove the seven miles in from his camp to say hello, and it was decided that we would all have dinner that night at the Miscoviches. This was decided because (1) the Fullertons always have dinner on Saturday night with the Miscoviches; (2) Johnny fires up his steam bath on Saturday nights, the only way the Fullertons can get a bath; and (3) down in the cook house, the steaks were already thawing.

We then went out to see the dredge in operation. The thing is over 30 years old. It is not a large dredge, as dredges go, but it looked large enough to me. The guys insisted that I should see the whole thing, and I, of course, had no objection. Seeing the whole thing involved being carried piggyback up and down ladders, inside and outside the dredge. My theory on this sort of thing is that if anyone is willing to carry me someplace new, then I am willing to be carried.

The dredge is operated on a 24-hour basis. As a piece of machinery, it could not have been simpler. Shovels on an endless belt dig up the creek bottom, carry it up about 30 feet, and drop it into sort of a shoot-the-shoot mechanism, which washes the gravel and sifts the gold out of it through various riffles onto cocoa matting where the gold becomes imbedded. It is an easy process because the gold is loose and because it is such an extraordinarily heavy metal. It is, you know, 35 times heavier than water.

The dredge is like an old beat-up Mississippi River boat, grinding and groaning and crunching its way up the creek. We stopped the dredge, scooped some of the sludge from between the riffles, put it in a pan with a little water, and there we were—panning for gold. I was allowed to keep what I panned. I have it still—a few little flakes of honest-to-God gold.

I was carried in a sort of modified fireman's carry—back, down the ladders, across the narrow gangplank, and through the mud to the pickup; then we drove into town.

Flat was founded in about 1910, with the discovery of substantial gold deposits in Otter Creek. There was a real gold rush, one of the last in Alaska. It is reported that, at the time, there were 10,000 people in Flat, but this is hard to believe. Certainly, for the first 30 years or so of its existence, Flat numbered between 3,000 and

5,000 in population and thus ranked as one of the larger cities in Alaska. The town has a current population of not more than 10 or 15 in the winter, with a few more added in the summer. Flat is about 250 miles from Anchorage, 300 miles from Fairbanks. In the early days, the only way of getting in and out of town was on foot in the summer and by dogsled in the winter. In its heyday, there was regular barge service up from the Yukon. Now, there is only weekly service by bush plane.

It seemed strange to see people in Flat. It looks so much like a ghost town that one gets a weird feeling when seeing actual inhabitants walking around through these decaying, fallen deserted buildings. The school house is as it was the last day of school, May 27, 1951. Open the door—there is not a lock in Flat—go inside, and there are the books, the desks, the old wood-burning stove made out of a petroleum drum. Children's drawings are pinned to the wall. George Washington and Abraham Lincoln's pictures are above the blackboard. Written on the blackboard is: "This is the last day of school. There may not be any school next year." There follows the signature of the teacher and her seven pupils.

Across the street is Tootsie's House. Tootsie was a famous Negro whore who lived in Flat for 40 years. Tootsie always served and sold liquor without a license, and, during prohibition years, ran the town's speakeasy. She was arrested during the 1920s for selling bootleg liquor by two revenue agents who barely got out of town alive. Tootsie was taken to Fairbanks and tried. They sought to make her turn state's evidence, telling her that if she would but give the names of the miners in the town who had built the still for her, she would go free. Tootsie refused resolutely, as she did all her life, to betray her friends and customers. She told the judge that, "All I know is I woke up one morning and there the liquor was." Tootsie got a year in jail. When she came back, she was welcomed with open arms.

Hugh Matheson's father and uncle lived in Flat off and on for 30 years, and they certainly must have known everyone in the town. Yet, Hugh says, when he came back from college and visited Tootsie's establishment for the first time, Tootsie said how pleased and honored she was to meet him. She said she had, of course, seen his father and uncle about town, but that as they were substantial and important men, she had never had the pleasure of meeting either gentleman—which, of course, says Hugh, was but another sign of Tootsie's loyalty.

Down the street is where Billy Burns lives. Billy is now in his 80s. I talked with him; he is as alert and as strong and healthy as a man in his 50s, certainly. The townspeople say that Billy has severe hypertension and that he has had it for over 40 years. For over 40 years, he has been expected to drop dead at any moment. There is talk of taking up a collection to send Billy back to Mayo's as a medical curiosity. He is much too nervous and high-strung to hold down a job now. In fact, he has been too nervous to hold down a job for more than 30 years! Yet, Billy chops all his own wood up on the mountainside, drags it down every year. He can still provide a fair share of his food by hunting. He survives largely on this and his social security check. He is, of course, a fairly sustained alcoholic; no one knows how or where the money comes from for his liquor.

Billy is a very argumentative man. He says that he has not spoken to half the people in town for over 20 years and that he can just barely stomach the remainder. In fact, he is thinking of moving to a cabin that he has up in the hills to get away from these " . . . interfering sons of bitches who keep sticking their noses into his business."

And then we went to call on Stella Parker. Stella is in her 70s; her husband died several years ago, and Stella now lives alone. She went Outside[1] last year to visit relatives in Seattle, and they clamped her in the booby hatch. It took her months to get out and back home to Flat, where everyone knows she is buggy, but they do not bother much about it. After all, Stella has always been buggy. She chops her own wood, and she now has a couple of deserted buildings full of brush, which she chopped last summer just to insure that, should the logs run out, she would still have something to burn. She is nervous about it, because, last year on March 17, it was 52 degrees below zero. She ran out of wood, and she got sick.

It was a harrowing experience for her, especially because she was flown out to a hospital in Anchorage. She is not going to let that happen again. Stella is Polish, and she is very big on the Blessed Virgin Mary. She spends a good deal of her time contemplating the myster-

---

[1]The term used by Alaskans for any place other than Alaska.

ies of the BVM, and she announced that she would begin praying for me. (This was entirely unsolicited.) Stella intends to pray for me every day for six months. She says her prayers are most efficacious. She has never failed yet, and in six months I am to write her and let her know how and in what way I am better. I thanked Stella and promised to write. Who knows?

We went back to the Miscoviches for dinner. The Fullerton brothers joined us. The Miscovich family used to have a large operation in Flat, and the mining camp is still run as it was then. We ate in the cook house, and we each had a huge steak, which was nicely cooked. There were biscuits and french fries and cookies and cake and helping upon helping of everything. As soon as night fell, of course, the temperature began to drop, and there was a nice feeling as the people would come stomping into the cook house, taking off their coats and hats, standing before the great wood stove to get warm. There was talk about old times and where people had gone, but there was also talk about current events. Everyone in Flat reads a great deal, for nights are long and winters are cold. The conversation was no less intelligent and really not very much less informed than at the average Washington dinner party. Everyone was interested in the election, especially in Bobby Kennedy's candidacy. There was spirited disagreement as to whether his running in a state not his own was a good thing.

After dinner and after the Fullerton brothers had their steam bath—a weekly Saturday night ritual—we drove out to the Fullerton camp on Willow Creek. This is a sluice box operation, run entirely by Rich and Jim Fullerton, with the assistance of one hired man. The hired man is a strange hermit, who is probably in his mid-30s. He has a black, shaggy beard; his hair is shaggy, likewise. He comes from Allentown, Pennsylvania, and apparently has an Ivy League education. He is thought of locally as some sort of a remittance man. He drives everyone in town up the wall by claiming he has been every place that is mentioned and has done any job that is discussed. He has lived in Flat for several years. He is a dark, morose sort of person, who used to go on two or three month binges, drinking night and day, drinking himself into a stupor. Since he began working with the Fullertons, however, he only gets drunk in a normal social sort of way, and people are really quite pleased with his rehabilitation. He has not left Flat in years, he used to hole up in his cabin all winter with a bottle. Last year, however, he bought a little snow cat, and now he spends the winter driving up and down the mountains.

The Fullertons, of course, grew up in Flat. They mine their holding every summer, and they winter in Seattle. Rich is married to, they say, a very nice wife. They have several children. She had already returned to Seattle by the time I arrived, so I did not have the opportunity of meeting her. Jim has never been married. He is somehow afraid of women. Jim lives with Rich and his family winter and summer, so it is as though he had a family of his own, anyhow. Jim is an accomplished accountant; Rich is an accomplished mining engineer. Together, they have been able to make gold-mining pay a pretty good living. Both of them are college graduates; both of them were in the service during the war. Neither of them expected to remain in mining or in Flat. They came back after the war to straighten out their affairs, and, somehow, they never left.

I spent the night sleeping in a little room off the cook house. When they asked me if I needed blankets, I said, "You're damned right I do." I told them how cold I get at night, so they fixed me up. They put a Canadian sleeping bag on my bed, one that is designed for sleeping outdoors in 60 degrees below zero weather. The thing was huge, filled with down, and heavy. Once I was in bed, I was imprisoned by the weight of it. I remembered that Charley Brown comic strip in which he puts on his coats and hat, his gloves and scarves and boots and things, and in the last picture he says, in a small voice, "I can't move." The bag was very warm; the air was clean and cold, and I fell asleep immediately. Getting up the next morning was like getting up at Oxford in my unheated room. There, of course, was no heat in the room; the day was cold and damp, and it was only strength of will that got me out of that bed.

The Fullertons, Matheson, Bobby, and Maury have all had extensive experience with Arctic winter. I got them to talking about their experiences, and it was fascinating. One thing I learned is that people really do dress for the cold. Although the temperature at Flat probably never got much below 15 degrees while I was there, the Flat residents were all wearing long woolen thermal underwear, down-filled jackets, and several layers of clothes. Sergi Agoff said that, when he was drafted and stationed at Fort Greely at Fairbanks, he was appalled at the skimpiness of the long underwear furnished by the Army.

They told me about an old Russian man, probably in his 70s, whom I later met. The previous summer, Flat had several days of real heat. One day, the temperature was recorded at 100 degrees. This old Russian drifted into camp, dressed as he always dresses—old coats, old shirts, old sweaters, old long underwear—sat down and said, "By God, if this hot weather continues, I'm going to take off my woolen underwear." He was still wearing his woolens.

This year has been a good berry year, so the bears have not been much of a problem. "Seen many bears in camp?" Rich Fullerton was asked. "Not a one," he answered. "What about that one you shot from the kitchen window?" asked his brother. Rich had forgotten about that one.

After breakfast, we went to inspect the Fullerton mining operation. It is most impressive and efficient. One brother runs the drag line; the hired man and the other brother run two cats. Between them, they have moved over 300,000 square yards of dirt this year. All this dirt is channeled into a sluice box where it is mixed with water and run down a series of riffles. The gold flakes drop out and are caught in cocoa matting. This matting is taken up, and the gold removed from it once or twice a year. When I was there, there was probably $60,000 or $70,000 worth of gold sitting out there in those mats.

We then drove over an incredibly bad road seven miles further, yet, to see the Agoffs. Their story is unique.

It all began about 40 years ago, when Harry Agoff, a wild Russian communist immigrant, began mining 14 miles outside of Flat. There has been a road to the Agoff spread only for the last two years. Until then, it was necessary to hike through the bush to get to their camp. Harry Agoff was a great drinker, who would come to town occasionally to argue and drink. He was by no means a stupid man. He began dating a schoolteacher, and she became pregnant by him. In those days of long skirts and corsets, etc., the school teacher actually kept her condition secret. She had the baby in the back room of the schoolhouse without telling a single soul in the town. Of course, when the town found out, it was incensed. The town forced Harry Agoff to marry the teacher, and that is how the Agoff family began. Harry took his teacher out to his camp and became, for all practical purposes, a hermit.

The firstborn child was a boy, and he was named Sergi. The second child was also a boy, and he was named Alvin. The boys were raised on the campsite. They were educated by their mother; they knew no other children; they have never had any formal education of any sort. They both still live on the campsite. Their father died several years ago; their mother still lives with them and cooks. This year, Sergi and Alvin have made about $100,000 clear. They will continue to make this kind of money for at least 15 to 20 years. They have found that kind of pay dirt. They mine it themselves, just the two of them. They have no hired help. Their overhead expenses are minimal. They are wealthy men.

They are also immensely strong men. I have never seen such solid muscles. They speak with a rather peculiar accent all their own. They speak slowly and thoughtfully. They read a good deal, and the books in their cabin are interesting: Marx, Engels, Thoreau, mining texts, and a variety of thrillers.

Sergi was drafted, and so was Alvin. Unfortunately, the day Alvin was inducted, he slipped in a shower and broke his ankle. He was released from service. As a result, he has never had the opportunity of living with people outside of Flat.

His brother, Sergi, did serve his two years in military service at Fairbanks. When he was released, he took a trip Outside to Seattle and the Northwest. He was riding on a bus up the coast, when he met a girl. When he got to Seattle, he stayed with the Fullertons. Hugh Matheson was also staying there at the time. Sergi announced he was going to marry the girl on the bus. Tremendous arguments ensued. "Jesus Christ, Sergi, you *can't*; you can't marry the first girl you ever met." Sergi thought it was a pretty good idea, though; and after several weeks of argument, he hunted down the girl, found her, asked her to marry him, and she accepted. She was a German girl who had worked a couple of years as a legal stenographer in Rio de Janeiro, and she was touring the United States before returning to Germany.

Instead of going home, she married Sergi on the spot and flew with him to Flat, hiked out through the bush, and took up housekeeping in the cabin. That was 15 years ago, and they are still married. They are very happy. Sergi did not know at the time he married the girl that she was of German aristocratic blood and that her family was very wealthy. As a result, Sergi and his wife spend a month or two every year in Germany. All the time they are there, they have the use of a Mercedes limousine and chauffeur; they go, too, to the Riviera. I am told that Sergi's in-laws are very fond of him, although in some ways they do not quite understand him. He has to be reminded not to buy a drink for the waiter at the same time he is buying a drink for himself and not to talk with the help as though they were his equal. None of this bothers Sergi very much; he does not consider it very important. He enjoys Europe well enough, but his heart is in Flat, and apparently his wife's heart is in Flat, too.

Of course, all of this has made Alvin desperately anxious to get married. It is almost beyond belief how hot he is to get married. So, Alvin a few years ago steeled himself and made the big effort. He went Outside. And he went for a ride on a bus. He rode on buses back and forth across the country; he rode buses for almost a month. "And," says Alvin, "Sergi, he got a wife, but all I got was pneumonia." He *did* get pneumonia, got on a plane, and flew straight back home to Flat.

I was trying to talk Alvin into coming back to Washington. I told him there were lots of girls back there. I promised to take him to lunch in the Senators' dining room. Alvin said, though, that he could not come. "Why not?" I asked. "You are a rich man, now. You ought to travel and see the world." Alvin replied that he had traveled. He had been Outside; he had been Outside for almost a month. Alvin was worried about the state of things Outside. "You know what? They're going to have to do something about those cars. They're getting out of hand."

One of Alvin's problems when he is Outside, or even in Anchorage—and he does go to Anchorage once or twice a winter—is that he tends to hit people. Alvin, and Sergi, too, believe that a man should be honest, kind, generous, and straightforward. If he is, they buy him a drink. If they meet a man who is not, they hit him in the face. This, of course, leads to various complications in societies more complex than their own.

Their cabin is a two-story log cabin. The logs came up the Kuskokwin and were dragged 50 miles from the river to the cabin site by the Agoffs and their dog team. The Agoffs are one of the few people in the area who still keep a dog team. Those dogs are big and mean. They do not like strangers, and they particularly do not like strangers in a wheelchair. The lead dog had little slitty brown eyes, and I would have shot him dead, had he not been on a chain. The Agoffs are making their own harnesses now because of the shoddy quality of dog team harnesses that are available in the stores.

In the cabin, they have an old upright piano. I was sitting beside it, and I happened to look down: there was a great big pot of something, a dull bronzy color. That something turned out to be $80,000 worth of solid gold.[2] Sergi was undecided as to what to do with it. They have already turned in $50,000 worth of gold this year. Someone told them that the tax people would take a big chunk of that $50,000 and would take an even bigger chunk of whatever additional gold they turned in. So, Sergi is thinking of burying some in the backyard. He would as soon have it in the backyard as in the bank. Should they have a bad year—say in 15 or 20 years' time—they would always be able to dig up the pot of gold in the backyard.

For almost 40 years, their father mined the headwaters of the creek. There was a great deal of overlay. The pay dirt was hard to get to; it was not particularly rich when they got to it. They never made much money, and there were many winters when they did not have enough to eat. Shortly before the old man's death, the brothers talked him into moving down the creek. To the great surprise of all concerned, the pay there was extremely good, and it looks like it will be good for many years.

We stayed for lunch and had an extremely good meal. There were the cookies and the cakes and the rolls and the biscuits and the usual things that show up on a table at Flat. The main course was

---

[2]The price of gold in 1964 was $35 an ounce.

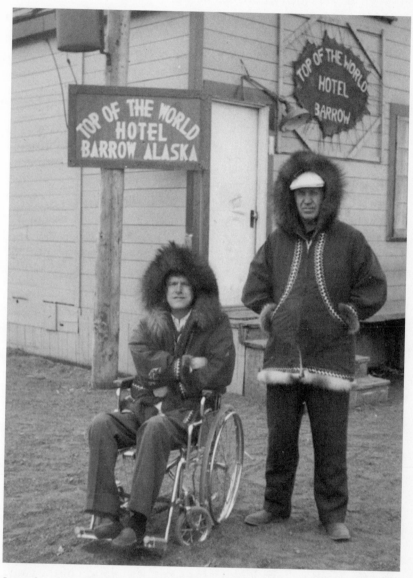

It may have been July, but at the Top of the World Hotel in Barrow, Alaska, in 1963, it was still cold. The hotel was the best hotel for 300 miles in any direction. The sanitary facilities consisted of a bucket with lye in the bottom.

ptarmigan that Alvin had shot the day before. It was very good. It tasted rather like dusky chicken, only not as dry.

When we were there, the Agoffs were getting ready for winter. They were bulldozing out a great big gully about a quarter of a mile above the house. They explained that this was, they hoped, going to divert a glacier, which in recent years had been encroaching on the house. The brothers and Sergi's wife spend the winters on the place, but their mother no longer does. "It's a hard winter out here," she said, "and so I winter in town." Town, of course, is Flat, and the Agoff house in Flat is about a half of a mile away from the other houses.

Sergi took me on a jeep trip up to the top of a roadless mountain. I must say, in spite of the hanging on I had to do to get up there, that the view from on top of the mountain was extraordinary.

Flat is set in a land of rolling hills interspersed with high snow-capped mountains. The tops of the hills were frosted, so that every tree and twig looked as though it had been dipped in ice. Driving through the hills was like driving through a forest of those strange, white Christmas trees they sell in supermarkets these days.

From the top of the mountain, you could look out in all directions. There is no one anywhere for mile after mile after mile—only moose and bear and wolves and foxes and, of course, the great herds of cari-bou, numbering into the thousands, which come through every year. (I saw a fox.)

Alvin is most interested in zoology and has read a good deal in the field, He would very much like to do some college work in it. However, he doubts that he could convince any college to take him, since he has no scholastic credentials of any sort. The family thinks that he would probably punch his professor in the nose the first time the professor asked him a question he could not answer. And he would probably be back in Flat before the first week was out.

The brothers hunt all year round, of course, and do not really worry too much about the game laws. Game wardens in Alaska fly in little planes. Every now and then, a little plane will come over and buzz the Agoff's camp, looking for signs of violation of the game laws. This spring, says Sergi, they had just finished skinning, cleaning, and hanging a caribou out of sight in the shed when one of the little planes flew over. It was a close shave, he said.

Conversation with these people in Flat was interesting. They remember conversations of years ago. They will say things like (to Matheson), "Hugh, you remember what you said to me in 1959, about how to build a riffle in a sluice box?"

Or they will say, "There was a man living down in Iditerod by the name of Charley Low, and he said in 1958 such-and-such."

It is as though they do not have too many conversations. Each one is carefully noted, its author recorded, and the facts sifted from it, filed away for future reference.

They welcome any man and give him hospitality simply because he is a man. They, in turn, expect to be well-treated by other men. They work very hard when they work, and they work most of the time. When they relax, they have a hell of a time. They, of course, drink buckets of coffee, buckets of liquor.

We drove back to town. By then Johnny Miscovich's son, Peter, had found the missing part to the airplane. It was then already getting dark, so we said good-by and flew back to Anchorage. The night was clear; there was a half-moon, and the snow-white mountains looked unearthly in the moonlight.

After we had landed, Bobby turned to me and said, "Well, the old crate worked pretty good. This was the first time I had ever flown it at night, you know, and I wasn't sure how the instruments were going to handle."

I hadn't known. We all went over to Bobby's house for a late dinner and some more drinks.

TIRED AND ANGRY

On the surface of things, my life looked hunky-dory. I was busy, useful, and popular. Beneath the surface things were different. In those days I did not know how different.

I find an early warning of this in a talk I made at the 1968 meeting of the President's Committee on Employment of the Handicapped. Looking back I see that I took my internal anger about my own situation and focused it outside myself onto the failings of society as a whole. Rather in the spirit of Rap Brown and Huey Newton, my anger certainly enlivened the proceedings.

WHEN THE BLACK POWER PEOPLE talk about burning down the cities, they are expressing the frustration they feel with the continuing hypocrisy and cant of a society which talks of ending injustice yet does nothing about it.

It is cruel to arouse expectations that are not fulfilled. It is not only cruel—it is dangerous.

Meetings such as ours, today, run the risk of arousing—yet again—the expectations and, unhappily, the frustrations of the handicapped.

For today we will hear the slogans of encouragement, the uplifting, heart-warming tributes to courage; we will give each other awards for hiring a "front office" cripple; we will pass resolutions and then it will be good-by for another year.

I, for one, am tired of it. I am bored with it all. I am angry.

For it is heartless. And cruel.

For many years, much has been promised the handicapped. I remember not so long ago a President declaring war, not only, he said, in behalf of the poor but in behalf of the handicapped as well.

How many hundreds of speeches, hundreds of committees, hundreds of meetings and tons and tons of good intentions have we had, and yet, here and now, in Washington, D.C. consider this:

I know a mentally restored college graduate with excellent qualifications who for over two years has tried to find a job in government. He has received every sort of excuse—all polite, all correct—but the fact is they are afraid of him and he has no job.

I know a young man who lives alone in a rented room in a city far from his home and friends. Confined to a wheelchair, he could drive a car but he cannot afford one. He could go to school if he had the proper counseling. He could hold down a job if he could find one. But he cannot and he lives alone—and bitter—on his welfare check.

The other day on the street in Southeast Washington I saw an adult black man in a wheelchair taking the sun in front of his apartment. He lived in public housing and there was a flight of steps at every entrance to his building. He could not get in, he could not get out, unless he was carried. That man could not be independent if he wanted to. The building, his home, his community, his society were stacked against him.

Last week I heard of a handicapped girl who lost her job because she was late returning from a vacation when an airline refused to carry her as a passenger.

I know a married couple, both in wheelchairs, with a young baby who had to look for months and months to find an apartment that was accessible to the chair and that would *accept* them as tenants.

These are personal examples. Let me point out three general examples:

New office buildings, new federal buildings continue to be constructed with such architectural barriers as steps and narrow doors that they might as well nail a sign on the door, "Crippled Keep Out."

The District of Columbia—unlike many large cities—still has no parking facilities or regulations whatsoever for handicapped drivers. So, even if the crippled does find himself a job in a building he can get into, chances are he still won't be able to get to park within a mile of his work.

As far as I know, there is no outreach program in the District of Columbia to find the crippled, determine their potential for rehabilitation, assist them in placement, and then follow through with personal counseling.

As far as I am aware, no one knows how many crippled there are, what condition they are in, what help they need, or how to get it to them.

The seriously crippled are really a very small minority. They need help on an individual basis. They need guidance, counseling and support, community by community, person by person.

Perhaps the government has a role to play. It seems to have a role in most everything these days. Primarily though it seems to me that this is a job for the voluntary local health agencies. This is what neighbors can do.

They *can* do it but they do *not* do it.

Do not talk to me of studies, of pilot projects. I have heard the speeches. I know all about the good intentions. Show me some action.

The violence in our cities has been ascribed to the frustrations caused by the failure to meet the rising expectations of the poor and the black.

I am here, today, to say that not only the poor or the black or the hillbilly are disadvantaged.

The crippled are, too.

Any Resemblance to Persons Living or Dead is Purely Coincidental

For more than 20 years, from the 1950s into the 1970s, I did not write about my disability. In fact, I worked very hard not even to think about it.

If people asked me—and many did—how I felt about my paralyzed body, I would reply, "Why I never think about it at all, not at all." And I honestly believed I was telling the truth.

In my Rhodes essay, I said I would ". . . let polio in only when it was impossible to keep it out." I was doing my very best to keep it out. Clearly, however, by the end of the 1960s, something was going wrong.

I did not know any disabled people nor did I want to. I might work in their behalf, give speeches, write articles, but I did not associate with them. Once, Senator Bartlett accepted an invitation to speak to a group of persons with disabilities, some of whom were severely crippled. At the last minute, he was unable to make the date so he asked me to fill in for him. I found it an agony: I was rigid with anxiety and hyperventilating. I thought I was going to pass out right there at the podium. It would be several more years before I understood something

*about the angry, passionate feelings this appearance caused me. These
feelings were not about their disabilities; they were about mine.*

*The late 1960s were an angry period and I was one of the angry
ones. Here is a fragment of something I wrote on the back of an United
Airlines folder in about 1968. It shows some of my ambivalence
towards disability:*

The Professional Handicapped

*I despise the handicapped banding together to form
groups or clubs for sports and social life.*

*This voluntary segregation serves to emphasize their
differences and is the antithesis to successful rehabilitation, which seeks adjustment to the disability and a
return to able-bodied society.*

*There is no more reason why one handicapped per-
son should know any others or associate with them or feel
any more responsibility for them than should a physically
fit person.*

*Physical disability is an accident and society's respon-
sibility to its less able is society-wide, not particular.*

*I must say in my own defense that I no longer hold such a view. In
fact, I have found much support and shared understanding from my
friends in the disability community. Our sense of togetherness is of
very great value to me.*

*The following are excerpts from a piece I wrote in the early 1970s
before my breakdown and depression. Today, reading it more than 20
years after it was written, I find myself shuddering and sad. I shudder
because my life really was like that; I am sad that I lived so many years
in such a state.*

*I do think that this is a remarkable piece of writing, but it is not
pretty. It is brutal and cold and angry. It depicts, all too accurately,
what my life was like.*

*Every one of the events described did take place, but not all at once.
Only the names and places have been changed to protect the innocent.
Even my name has been changed from "I" to "he."*

*There is something very curious about this piece. It is very long, and
the obvious honesty and care with which it was written show that it*

was not written quickly. It contains several of my carefully worked-out theories on disability. And, yet, I do not remember writing it. I had forgotten it completely. I found it in an old trunk in the garage. The mind does remarkable things. It forgets what it cannot bear to remember— unbearable pain, for example. Perhaps that is what happened here.

I need only add that, since I wrote this piece, I have learned a trick or two about drinking on airplanes. I can now do it without worrying!

"DAMN THEM ALL, damn them all, damn them all to Hell."

"I am going to make it in their world. I am going to make it." His anger was fear. He was angry at the unfairness of his predicament. He was angry to cover his fear, a fear caused by his utter helplessness and dependence. Like Odysseus, his only weapon was his cunning; his only comfort, his anger. He would use both, and damn them all.

It was going to be all right. The plane was making its approach to La Guardia. People were gathering their things, reaching their coats from the overhead racks, interested only in themselves and getting off the plane as quickly as possible. They didn't stare at him, they didn't even notice him. They just used their full bodies in an unconscious flaunting of their ability to cope physically with—with what? With the plane, their lives, earth, gravity. Whatever it was, it was still a sweet and hard sight for him.

Two years before he had been one of them; but now he was not. Then, he could stand and run and take pleasure in his body. But then, of course, he was as unaware of the value of his body and what it could do as his fellow passengers were now. They, bust with their own interests, were unaware that he was watching them with envy and awe, fear and hostility. Whatever the end of this flight and the resumption of his truncated life might bring, he would never be one of them again.

His legs were paralyzed, totally. He had no trunk muscles and sat upright only because a canvas brace kept his backbone erect. His muscles were of varying degrees of strength, strong enough to pull himself from his wheelchair into a car or chair. The operation was a slow business, involving inching along what was euphemistically called a slideboard. After months of practice, he could do it in only a matter of several minutes and he could do it himself—a source of personal satisfaction and perhaps a promise of independence.

Independence had assumed a dreadful importance. The onset of the disease when he was 20 had brought with it a series of shocks. A young man, proud of his physical and sexual powers, his appeal and his future, found these things gone. They were broken, wiped out, gone forever and forever. They would *never* be back. His mind, proud and ambitious, was still there; but the body, the means of serving his pride and ambition, was gone. In its place was the curious soft, pudgy body of a baby—fully as helpless and as pink but lifeless. His body just lay there. He could feel it—and for a long time, he had felt severe physical pain. He could see his leg; he could try to control it, to direct it, to move it, to turn to one side or another, but nothing would happen. His mind had lost its control of his body. His body no longer answered any authority of his. It was dead, and by some fantastic joke, he was not. Instead, he was on an airplane coming into La Guardia, just like the other passengers.

He looked about him: It was doubtful that even one or two of the other passengers was aware that he was crippled. He had on his suit, a clean shirt and tie. His hair was cut, his face clean. The fact that his hands shook as he read his magazine would have been noticed only by someone closely observant—and there was none close to observe. The stewardess had made sure of this by putting a "reserved" pin on the seat next to him, so that no one would experience the possible embarrassment of sitting beside him. "You will be more comfortable, won't you, honey?" asked the stewardess, a question he considered bald in its hypocrisy.

The flight was going to be all right. He had not slept the night before, he had not slept that morning, in fearful anticipation. He had taken a double phenobarbital, but it was going okay. His therapist had driven him from the protection of the rehabilitation center to the airport with plenty of time to spare. He had left the car with the help of the slideboard by himself. His therapist was pleased. The airlines had been informed that he would be on the flight, and, as it originated in the city, he was boarded early. This meant that, before the other passengers were at the gate, his wheelchair was placed on a

pallet forklift and raised to the level of the plane entrance. His therapist had wheeled the chair into the plane. As his parents had paid for
a first-class ticket, there was space for his chair in front of the bulk-
head seat. He was able in a minute or two of effort, with the help of
his slideboard, to edge himself over into the seat. They took the board
and the chair away, and the trip began.

The flight had been, as they say, uneventful. To him, this meant
that he had controlled his bladder and did not have to piss. For, if he
had, he could not have. His wheelchair was stowed away somewhere
in the belly of the plane, and the washroom was at the end of the aisle.
There was no way whatever of getting out of his seat to the toilet,
and just the knowledge of the fact made his bladder nervous and his
penis have a spasm of anxiety. He had drank no fluids since the night
before, and his kidneys literally were dry: he had nothing to pee,
and, anyway, the flight was over.

"We'll wait till everyone's out. All right, honey?" the stewardess
asked, or rather reported; and the other passengers filed by, down
the steps, into the evening rush hour of New York. He could see, at
the gate, passengers to Boston waiting to board the plane as it continued its flight.

He waited. Nothing happened, although he heard discussion.

"We have an Invalid Assist. Where's the chair?"

"No one told us you had an I.A."

"Atlanta did not get a chair—will you?" Her voice was not pleasant.
This is the end of my run, and I can't leave until all my passengers
leave; and he is one of my passengers. Get him out.

Still nothing happened. Five minutes later—five hours it seemed—
the agent arrived with a wheelchair. It was not his. It was an airport
wheelchair, and the arms were not detachable. He did not think that
he could use his slideboard to get into this chair.

"Where is my slideboard?" he asked the agent.

"What's a slideboard?" asked the agent of the stewardess.

"It's a piece of wood he sits on," said the girl. "I think they checked
it or something."

One of the things about being crippled, he had noticed, was that
people did not talk to you or with you, but about you. It was as
though you were deaf, as well as paralyzed.

"I can't get out of this chair without it," he said, and he was ashamed to say it. It hurt him to say it, and he said it lowly.

"Can he get into the chair?" the agent asked, and as he answered by shaking his head, the agent went on to the stewardess, "You should have let us know, for God's sake. This is a full invalid assist. He can't get down the steps or *anything*."

More men were called, and he was lifted into the strange wheelchair. They dropped one of his legs. And they strapped him in, because regulations said he had to be strapped in. It made him feel like he was being ordered off the plane in a strait jacket.

They carried the chair down the steps wrong. He tried to tell them so: "Tilt the chair backwards, over its rear axles, and one man can roll it down the steps."

The agent, barely older than he was and already harassed and no doubt embarrassed, was having no more advice from anyone; was, in fact, treating his passenger like some inanimate man doll that, through some practical joke, had become his responsibility to dispose of. They went down the steps backwards. It took four men a good deal of effort to control the chair, and he felt neither happy nor even secure as he went down the steps, head first, with his body raised higher than his head.

The Boston passengers watched the proceedings with the detachment of TV viewers. Adult strangers stare at the breed, he thought, without compassion, without passion, without interest. They are not rude; they simply block out completely the very existence of the crippled. Children who have not yet learned self-protection were often rude, blunt in their questions, but seldom without compassion.

Once inside the gates, his parents were waiting, proud and happy to have him back. He had gone to the rehabilitation center on a private railroad car, flat on a stretcher, with nurses and oxygen tanks in attendance. No plane or train would take him. It was only because of his father's money and mortgaging the house, again, that he had been able to afford the trip down and the years of treatment. His parents had wanted to come down and fly back with him to see that he was all right. But the time must come for him to learn to walk in the world by himself. And, even though the language had no substitute for the verb walk to express what he must do, he felt the time had come to do it. He would not, in spite of the best of intentions of some, the lack of interest of others—in spite of fortune, fate, and folly, he would not spend his life in the upstairs bedroom.

And this time was as good as any to curse the fates, gamble disaster, and do the very simple thing white, middle class Americans do almost daily: take the plane trip and take it alone.

Alone he was determined to be. He was crippled; he was handicapped, but he was going to attain his independence. He was always going to be helped; he would never be able to climb stairs or walk. His strength would always be limited, and he would always be confined to a wheelchair. Confined, he thought, was descriptive. Like a lion in the zoo, he would be caged for life in his wheelchair. Physically dependent, he would, at least, or die, attain independence of mind and mood.

To start with, even this would not be easily achieved. At the height of his illness, he was mentally dependent, too, on his parents. Or absorbed by them, or, like a healthy man linked in blood transfusion to a sick man, his parents' determination and love and will for his life had been pumped into him. At his sickest, he had not given a damn about his life or its continuance. There was very little left to continue. The machines expanded his lungs to bring the air in and contracted them to push it out. The machines fed him through tubes and extracted his wastes through tubes. All the processes were kept going; and, in spite of his temperature, his infections, his discomforts, his pain, life kept on.

During those nights of dreadful pain, death was like a cool cave on a summer's day, a retreat only a few steps away, a place he could go, now, easily, just by deciding that enough was enough—he would have no more. It was never fearful; it was comforting, if anything.

Yet, through this strange transfusion, this deep entanglement with his parents' will for him to live, and because of a strong desire not to disappoint or hurt them at this time, when they were totally and openly exposed in their love for him, he never went into the cave, although he stood many times at its entrance.

The cave had receded; the convalescence had begun, leaving him whole in mind, but not in body. It had also left him with this fierce desire to be independent of others. It was as though, perhaps, he resented the bonds that his parents' love had placed on him at that critical point. He had lived *for* them and not by his own choice. At the critical point, he had no choice. He would not get in that position again. He would not let his ties, his obligations, his loves become so strong as to influence such a decision again.

While this is what had happened, and this is how he had reacted, he thought of his independence in a much simpler manner: he wanted to be an individual human being, a man in his own right. He did not want to be somebody's dependent. He would not live off his parents, and he would have his own life, to the best of his ability. He put it in his own thinking that he would be as much like other self-reliant grown-up men and women as possible.

But, by then, to him, the breaking of family ties was something very different than the average man coming of age: severing the ties of youth, replacing them with ties of love, marriage, and new family.

By then, already, although he did not know it, the struggle to escape the obligation placed on him by his family's love was not at all like the average cycle. Not at all. He was coming to fear love—all love—and the demands it made. He feared love, because it had kept him alive. It had narrowed his choice, when he most needed it, and was responsible for his life and gave him no guide on how to live it.

He would not be so trapped again.

His parents met him, their grown son, at the gate; and he was pleased to see them, beyond his ability to say, and far beyond his desire to let on. His father found his bags, his slideboard, and his wheelchair. His father, in public, lifted him into his own familiar wheelchair. He was relieved and exhausted. In the hubbub of La Guardia, at 6:00 p.m., he was not noticed: he was ignored, and, thus, almost back in the protective privacy of known people and places.

They went out to the taxi ramp, his mother pushing the chair, his father with the bags. At once, he was assaulted by sight and sound. The scene was brilliant, black and white, as if lit by flash bulbs and spot lights. The noises were crashing, harsh, strident. He found himself surrounded by yelling people, horns blaring, doors slamming, engines revving. Loud and physical. There were too many people, too few taxis. There was no line, and people were fighting for the attention of the taxi dispatcher and the cabs he had found for them. People pushed into the cabs, almost before the arriving passengers had time to push out. It was a situation in which he was hopeless to compete, and he thanked God his parents were there to compete for him. He held his shoulders back, his head up. His neck was skinny; so were his hands. He held his slideboard in his lap.

After 20 minutes of waving and shouting, his father and the dispatcher got a cab. He rolled up to it and was dismayed to see it was a Checker Cab with seats high above the ground—higher by far than the seats of other cars. He did not know whether he could possibly get into the cab on his slideboard; he did not think so. The board angle would be at least 45 degrees. It would slip out, and he would fall, Even if he could make it—it would take a long time. His hands were already wet. His vision became slightly dazed in the lights, and the noise sounded more harshly. He held his head up and remembered that he was handsome and that he could make people like him, or he used to be able to.

The dispatcher reached for the door, but the cab driver was too quick for him. The cabby slammed down the door locks.

"God damned if I'll take any damn cripple," he said.

He did not look happy about it. The dispatcher shouted at the driver; the driver shouted back. "I'll get your number," shouted the dispatcher, exasperated, angry. "Regulations, you've got to take him. What are you, some sort of a creep?"

The driver sat immobile within his sealed cab, staring rocklike ahead, unmoving. Strangers began shouting, berating the driver. His father argued. Some people on the other side of the cab began rapping on the window.

"If you won't take him, take us. Well, you just can't let a cab get away," one of them said to the crowd, as they got into the now-unlocked cab and rode away.

It did not take long, the whole thing. It was over in seconds. Yet, to him, it seemed very long. To him, it seemed not only now, not only here and now, but for a long time, for years and years ahead. At one point, he said, or tried to say, to his father, "Let's get away. Let's go away; we can come back later," he said, "We can come back." But his father did not pay attention. He sat still, staring straight ahead, fearing everything forever at this, his homecoming. He held his head high with a certain winning smile forlornly on his lips.

"That cabby is a God damn creep," the dispatcher told the crowd. "How would he like to be a cripple? It might happen to him some day, you know. He might be a cripple, too."

But then the dispatcher forgot about it, and the crowd forgot about it. The crowd charged, and they were too busy fighting for their cabs to notice him.

His father found another cab, and there was not time for the slideboard, what with the honking and all. His father lifted his grown son, like a baby, into the cab, and they went home.

He was 22.

★ ★ ★

Years later, he was in New York for the day. The limousine was waiting for him as he came out the door of Alfred Dunhill. He had arranged for time to stop here before returning to La Guardia. He paid $80 for a new collar for his dog, an absurd amount, but it was his dog and his money. In point of fact, he had nothing else to do with the money.

Getting in the car was tiring. As the years moved by, he found his arm muscles and his body tiring more quickly and taking much longer to recover from fatigue. He felt, at times, they never really recovered, that each strain upon them diminished his strength by that much, and that there would come a day in the months or years ahead when they would fail to function at all. He would just lie on his bed, alive and helpless.

His driver held the wheelchair in place. With the front door open, he inched his body forward on the wheelchair seat. With his left arm, he placed his limp left foot and leg into the car. Then, with his right arm grasping the little rain gutter above the door, he pulled the trunk of his body into the car and his right leg along after, as a separate operation. He sank back gratefully into the luxury of the seat as his driver collapsed the chair and stowed it in the trunk.

"It's not getting any easier," a friend had said to him at lunch. No, it wasn't, he thought; it certainly wasn't. His life was as structured and false as a movie star's. The star's makeup and glamour, the tinsel that surrounds the star, was planned; the star's appearance in public arranged for full effect. Inevitably, time would eat away at such stardom: the makeup would take longer, as reality sank farther and farther from the public image. Just so in his life, he too wore a sort of makeup: he had worked very hard over the years to become a certain *sort* of person with a handicap. This person was the cheerful but not saccharine, confident but not cocky, direct, but not bitter, sort of person. He had become the person who accepts his handicap comfortably and, thus, makes others comfortable in its presence. He had accomplished this person by consciously projecting a secure self reliance. When with him, people sensed they need not fear that he would burden them with his responsibilities. His mental state and physical condition were not contagious. He had learned early on that, no matter how kind, well-meaning, or determined another might be, he could or would not bear to assume a part of the real burden of being crippled. People flee from a sick room, leave their corpses on the battlefield, and prefer not to see their crippled neighbors. He often thought how much happier they would be if we were kept like lunatics in lunatic asylums or lepers in leprosariums. The price he paid to live in the world of the fit was to keep his burdens and his bitterness to himself. He tried—whether with friends, employees, or strangers—to be cheerful, healthy, interested, and never dependent or vulnerable. This makeup he assumed, like the movie star, but time was eating away at it. His life had become no easier.

Yet, in the material sense, it had, indeed, become easier: limousine and driver in New York, a handmade sports car waiting for him at the other end of the shuttle, a new home built and designed at his direction for his comfort and convenience, a housekeeper to worry about the house, secretaries and assistants to attend him at the office, a dog. He had no responsibilities: no family, no parents, no children, no wife. His life was under his control alone. It brought him no happiness, but he had never expected happiness. Happiness had been killed along with hope, illusion, enthusiasm, and anticipation over a quarter of a century ago that week at college when polio caught him.

Material comfort made his life more pleasant. Financial independence made his life more bearable. True, he still dreamed of penniless paralysis in an old man's home, but each year this condition became less likely. He had set out to neutralize his handicap with his pleasant looks and easy personality and to use his brain to build a reputation and earn the money he needed for his independence. He had succeeded in his plan, and the reputation and money were growing.

At La Guardia, his driver wheeled him to his flight gate. The attendants knew that he was coming. He came to New York almost every week, and the procedure was invariable. They tagged his wheelchair "escort," which meant it would be put last in the baggage compartment when they left and brought from the belly of the plane up to him in his seat in the cabin when they arrived. Seat 1-B, first class, had been reserved, the only seat to which he could transfer from his wheelchair without assistance. He was preboarded, his wheelchair stowed away before the others came on board. He was always pleased by this service. Even after 25 years, he was still self-conscious about strange people and crowds, especially when he had to do something that stretched the limit of his muscular powers, like transferring from chair to seat. He knew how strangers would watch, but not watch, pretend he was not present. He knew, too well, the thrill of embarrassment and horror that spread through a crowd if he should fall from the chair as he was transferring or, even worse, be catapulted out of his chair should something jam his front wheel.

Because strangers were shocked and horrified, he was embarrassed even more. Falling out of his chair was a frightening thing because he lacked the strength to break the fall. He had fallen in various situations and surroundings—some of them absurd, some funny, but all of them intimate and personal. Most people avoid fighting in public, going naked, or otherwise exposing their vulnerability. So, too, would he pray that if he were to fall, he would do so in private. Later, after the fall, he could make jokes about it—to put others and himself at ease—but, when it happened, the jokes were far away.

Although he was resigned to his condition and would not allow himself to envy others, he could not help but look on them with wonder. He could not stand going to the beach for the very beauty of the whole young healthy body was intoxicating and dangerous to his mental defense. Now, as he watched the passengers filing down the aisle, he was filled again with awe. Each and every one had systems that worked: hearts that pumped, lungs that filled, legs that moved. Surely, some must have been as deadly tired as he, some as worried, tense, or frightened. The sale of tranquilizers and laxatives surely indicated that his condition and his complaints must be fairly close to universal. But, if so, where were they? The human ability to hide the horror of life, to suffer the real and unreal ailments, to keep going and to keep it from each other, knew no limit. They filed down the aisle looking just like anyone else. For that matter, he thought, no doubt I look just like anybody else, seated here in the airplane.

But he did not, and the thought made him yearn for a drink—a drink he could not allow himself on an airplane. Drinking beer or Scotch always ran the risk that he would have to urinate, and this would clearly be impossible.

He *did* look different. In spite of the money he paid his tailor, his legs were small and withered and looked it. His hands especially were skeleton-like and trembled as they struck a match or held a cigarette. His body was a funny shape, pear-like, in spite of the corset back brace which he wore. Here again, there was nothing much you could do about it—even though, as he so often thought, the aesthetics of it all were painful to him. He waited for the plane ride to be over; he was tired. He stared ahead and thought of the day and its business, and of tomorrow and its business, and of the next day's business. His business was more important to him than any games or puzzles or television. It filled his thoughts, and for this, he was often grateful.

Just before the plane was landing, he gave the stewardess his escort baggage claim check, so that she could hand it to the station agent, who would be at the end of the terminal jetway as the plane came to its gate. This time, he noted with some alarm, the plane was not taxiing to its usual berth at gate 10. Indeed, it stopped away from the jetways, and a flight of stairs was wheeled up to the airplane door.

"Jesus Christ," said the station agent, as he first peered in the cabin. "Why didn't they tell us there was someone in a wheelchair on board? It's two o'clock in the morning. How am I going to find porters at this time of the night to carry him down these stairs?"

The agent was angry. But trapped in his airplane seat, he was angry too. This would be an assault on his dignity. His legs, waist, and chest would be strapped into one of those narrow aluminum chair-like carts that the airlines use for carrying the infirm up and down stairs and up and down the aisles of airplanes. He preferred, in fact, being carried in arms by one of the baggage men or the agent. He only weighed slightly over 100 pounds, and the fuss and bother of being so carried, the spectacle, were considerably less embarrassing.

Airlines, however, had decided in recent years the danger of legal suits was so great that strict procedures must be instituted; this policy meant always the aluminum straitjacket chair. In spite of the late hour and the difficulty of finding assistance, it only took 15 minutes after the other passengers had disembarked before he, too, was in the terminal. This was 15 minutes longer on the job for the stewardess and the station agent, too, but they took it reasonably well.

He was pleasant and cheerful, thanking them for taking the time and going through the additional bother that his handicap had caused them. He did not feel very much like thanking them—he was tired and it was late, and there was really no excuse for taking 15 minutes to unload him and his chair from the plane—but he did so because he knew there would be other times, other nights, when he or some other handicapped person would cause healthy people some unexpected and unlooked-for burden. It is one of the obligations of the handicapped to be meticulous in thanking people for little favors. Like alpine cabins that overnight hikers must clean up before leaving so they will be clean for the use of the next hikers to come along, the handicapped must try by their actions to leave pleasant memories as they pass through so that, when crippled travelers come through in future days, clerks, ticket agents, and bellhops will treat them kindly. The "little favors," as they appear to normal people, are, in fact, of "make-or-break" importance to the crippled. To help a wheelchair up a curb, to turn a key in the lock for an arthritic hand, to guide a blind man to his door may be Boy Scout deeds, but they save the self-respect of the crippled person. This is why the crippled must be gracious and clearly appreciative. There is no guarantee whatsoever that the fit need continue to give the help upon which the handicapped are so dependent.

After 25 years, he had found that these favors were given only when they cost no sacrifices. This was why he had worked so hard to gain such physical independence as he had. This was why he had worked to obtain his money and position. Money could not buy his physical independence, but it could buy physical assistance on which he could count. There was a difference—a substantial difference, he knew—between the reliability and relationship between a chauffeur hired to drive you to work each morning and a neighbor who volunteers to assist you in time of need. He first learned something of this when he returned to work. There were five steps into the building in which his office was located. The first several mornings, people were kind, assisting him up the steps. After the first week or two, he noticed the same people tended to use other entrances into the building in order to avoid the effort.

He had always thought of this effect as the parade syndrome. He once was in a crowd, waiting for a parade to pass. People were most kind, clearing a path for his wheelchair right up front so that he could see the President and his party as they drove past. At the moment, however, that the President drove past, the crowd became so enthusiastic, it surged forward, completely enveloping his chair and blocking his view entirely. There was, he had decided, nothing nasty about such behavior; it was thoughtless, but not ill-intentioned. It was, simply, just the way it would always be.

Driving out, skirting the city along the river and then through the woods to the small house that was his, the solitary singular house in the woods that was his, he was taunted once again by the warmth and promise of the summer night. There was no other car on the road. He had the cheap joy, as, driving with the hand controls, he took his sports car up to 80, 85, 90 miles an hour. The air with its balm pushed through the cab of the car, and there was no one else who knew what his life was like.

There was no one he knew, nor would he ever allow, again, anyone the chance to try. The loneliness of the wooded road came upon him, and he was glad that his dog and his house were waiting for him. He turned off the car motor and placed the automatic shift into park. Carefully, he inched his way across the console separating the driver's seat from the other front seat. Once on the other seat, he lifted his legs, one by one, by gathering up the trouser material at the knee, pulling the leg over the console.

He opened the door. With his left arm braced and his left hand firmly holding the metal ledge under the dashboard, he turned in his seat. He pulled the back of the front seat forward and held it forward with his chin and upper right arm. With his right hand, he backed the wheelchair out of the back seat, big wheels first, onto the driveway. Still balanced by his left hand under the dash, he turned back in his seat, and, with his right hand, spread open the folding wheelchair on the pavement beside the car and locked its wheels.

Before getting out of the car, he checked, as always, to make sure he had the car keys, that the removable wheelchair arm was within easy reach, and that his briefcase and package were reachable as well. He then worked his way into the wheelchair, put its detachable arm back in place, took his briefcase and package. He was home.

BLACK BIRD

Da steht auch ein Mensch und starrt in die Höhe,
Und ringt die Hände vor Schmerzensgewalt;
Mir graust es, wenn ich sein Antlitz sehe—
Der Mond zeigt mir meine eigne Gestalt.

A man stands there too, staring up,
And wringing his hands in anguish;
I shudder when I see his face—
The moon shows me my own form.

"Der Doppelgänger"
HEINRICH HEINE

As the last piece makes crystal clear, I was in heavy emotional trouble. My anger and grief over my condition, and my twisted self-pity were leading me towards a black hole. This hole was to prove as painful as polio—if not more so.

Below is an account of my clinical depression and how I got out of it. It was difficult to write, and I do not intend to write about it again. I wrote the piece in 1975 and publish it only now.

IT STARTED ON MY 40TH BIRTHDAY in October 1972. Friends had a surprise party for me out at our favorite restaurant in the country. Because of the rigors of Washington social life, it was not really a surprise because the day had to be arranged to suit everyone's calendar. Ten or twelve of my friends were there. It is difficult to be more accurate—the party was three years ago, and already, names and faces are hazy. In the Washington I know, few stay very long. They are here for a year or two with the embassy or the paper, or here on home assignment, and then they are off again. It's a world of new friends and farewell parties. The girl I was going with at the time was there. That couple we saw so often that year was there and so was a couple from the office.

We were late, the others had already arrived. Conversation flowed easily. We laughed and drank, and it was like all Washington dinner parties.

Then, quite suddenly, it wasn't. It was my 40th birthday. For the very first time in my life, and quite suddenly, I realized that youth was past and old age was not far distant. This was no great vision. Everyone grows up. Everyone gets old. Everyone dies. I knew that. But for one brief moment, I could feel it, really *feel* it. High above the table, a giant black buzzard flapped its wings, and I was frozen with fear. The moment passed. I opened my presents and received, among others, a homemade necktie and a jar in which to keep sticks of macaroni. It was a nice party, but as I recall, it was the beginning of the end.

A few months later in January, I flew to Alaska to give a speech. The occasion was the opening of a treatment center for crippled persons in Anchorage. This was a center in which I had taken a good deal of interest. Volunteers had worked hard and raised much money to provide high-quality treatment and caring in a region which hitherto had provided no treatment of any sort. This was no ordinary occasion and, for my part, I wanted to give no ordinary dedication speech.

I am myself badly crippled as the result of a childhood case of polio. Although not deformed, I am paralyzed from the waist down and confined to a wheelchair. This has not hindered me in my career. I have held high-level jobs in the Executive Office of the President and on Capitol Hill. At the time of the speech, I was director of the

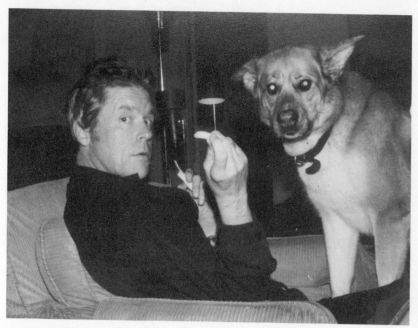

During my depression, my dog Dusty often stood protective guard over me throughout those miserable months.

Washington office and chief lobbyist for one of the seven largest oil companies in the world. I did free-lance writing as a hobby, had recently finished my second book, and was planning my third. To all appearances, my life was one of achievement, balance, and satisfaction. I had been asked to give the dedication speech at the treatment center because I had helped with lobbying and fund-raising.

On the flight out, I thought about the Center and the speech. The Center, I felt, meant a good deal to crippled Alaskans and not just because of the treatment offered. It was important to the crippled as a visible symbol that the people of Alaska cared about them. An effort had been made to accept them into the family of society and not hide them away as embarrassment hidden away in an upstairs bedroom. I wondered if all the good people who had worked to make the Center possible understood this. And then, I wondered if they understood what it felt like to be crippled.

I resolved that I would try to tell them, in my speech.

The flight is a long one, even by jet. There was plenty of time to think in that congenial isolation of the sky. Although I had given many speeches, I had never spoken about being crippled. In fact, I had thought very little about the subject. It was just there—a given, as other people have big noses or red hair—I was crippled. So, it was necessary to dig hard to find out in fact how I did feel about it. In the process, I had to ask myself questions I had never asked before. The answers were forthcoming and became the basis of what I felt would be a good speech, perhaps even a gripping one.

The speech was well received. You could hear a pin drop as I spoke. I was given a standing ovation. It was of interest that the three or four handicapped people in the audience made a special point of telling me how moved they had been. As I remember, the substance of the speech was that throughout history cripples had been hidden away. Crippled people were, I said, a visible and unpleasant reminder of the frailty of every man. And, therefore, I said, the sight of the crippled induced a certain fear and loathing amongst the physically fit. As a crippled person, I could testify that this fear and this loathing were sensed by the crippled and that it served to enforce their own burden of guilt and self-loathing. Therefore, I said, the treatment center was far more than a building. It was a gesture from the fit to the crippled. It was a gesture that said we cripples belonged; we, too, had a place in the community.

It was at some point in this admittedly gritty message that it happened again. As at my 40th birthday, it lasted but a moment, but the warning was unmistakably clear. At some point in the speech, I suddenly and immediately and totally *felt* the meaning of the speech I was giving. For the first time in my life and for only a split second, I realized how I felt about being crippled, about living in the world of the fit. High above me, the black bird flapped its wings. And for that split second, I was consumed by a passion so dreadful as to shatter my whole being. I did not know whether I could continue the speech or, indeed, whether I could continue my life. But I did continue, and, as I say, the speech seemed well received.

My depression began that spring. I did not know what it was. I had never experienced such a thing, and I did not record its advance. I was terribly tired, and sleep did not refresh. In fact, I could not sleep—whole nights would pass without sleep. Once or twice, I went nights at a time with no sleep. I was frightened all the day, terrified at night, fearful of being alone, unable to answer the phone, incapable of not answering it. My muscles ached with tension, my hands shook; my neck was so stiff I could look neither left nor right. I could not read for the words danced in front of my eyes; I could not write for my right hand, even when guided by the left, would only function erratically. Food had no taste, paintings no color, music no charm. I did not seem able to tell anyone what was wrong, nor was there anyone who seemed able to offer me solace.

And all this time, I was working—working, in fact, on a major and sensitive project and maintaining an active social life at night. It was, after all, part of my job to entertain and to attend the receptions, cocktail parties, and dinners of official Washington. I had never been a heavy drinker but I found to my surprise, that large amounts of alcohol and boisterous talk would ward off for a few hours the fears and fatigue I was experiencing. Considering the amounts of barbiturates I was consuming to sleep—or not to sleep, often enough—it is surprising the combination of drugs and alcohol did not kill me. There were many nights I wished that it would.

This sort of life continued until one morning in June. After a night, sleepless and terror-filled, I found myself unable to get up. After much struggle and painful effort, I finally managed to get myself dressed, but I was unable to leave the house. I spent the day seated in the old black, leather morris chair, which had been my great-grandfather's. I neither stirred nor spoke, so great was my depression. The great black buzzard sat heavy on my shoulder. It would not go away.

Words are poor things. Direct description cannot approach the experience of acute depression. Analogy fails. I only say from personal experience that the pain of acute paralytic polio in no degree equaled the agony and despair, the abject helplessness of depression.

After three weeks, I was sufficiently recovered to return to work. For the remainder of the year, I struggled with my problem. Sometimes I was better, sometimes better for weeks at a time, but always the depression lurked at the back of my mind to reappear if I left an evening unplanned, a moment unscheduled. I was ever on guard.

Throughout that year, I continued to operate, to work, to entertain. Once, after a dinner with the company's deputy chairman, who had flown in from London, I caught an unexpected glimpse of my face in a mirror. It was gaunt, and the eyes were glazed with tears. I was not crying. I could not cry. So great was the strain of keeping up my guard that tears were forced from the eyes as they are when a man strains to lift a great weight. Every phone call, meeting, business lunch, or dinner produced this strain.

The Christmas holidays were dreadful; artificial gaiety enforced by absolute, rigid self-control. Once they were over, the full depression returned with the dreary rains of January. I had struggled a solid year with this depression, and, at last, I broke.

Broke may not be the right word. What may be more correct is to say that, at last, at long, long last, I made a decision to do something about my condition. But, again, this is inaccurate. In the helpless despair of my illness, I was incapable of deciding whether I wanted cream in my coffee. I was at that point unable to take any step or decision of importance. Nevertheless, I did get myself to a psychiatrist.

The appointment was for eight o'clock in the morning so as not to interfere with my business day. It was the year of the oil embargo, and the morning was as black as midnight. A freezing rain was falling, and I had neither raincoat nor umbrella. The doctor's office was in his home, and he had agreed to meet me outside to pull my wheelchair up the two steps of his stoop. He thought I would honk my car horn as I arrived and I thought he would look outside for me at eight, no horn.

For a year, I had refused psychiatric help. I did not believe in it. It was hocus-pocus nonsense. In truth, I was scared of it. Not scared so much of a man called a psychiatrist, but scared, rather, of opening chambers in my head better left unopened, of releasing passions— similar to the ones I had felt at the treatment center speech—which were far too destructive to be released. I am of Irish heritage, and as one of my relatives said, "We Irish don't go to psychiatrists; we drink whiskey. Have another." The combination of depression and fear made it very hard for me to get my wheelchair out of the car that morning into the icy rain.

And then, the doctor did not open his door. Rush-hour traffic drowned the sound of my calls to him. I sat in the curb in front of his house, wet, freezing, helpless, and impotent for 15 minutes, waiting. I could not go back for now, truly, with the depression upon me again, there was nothing to go back to. The end, foreshadowed at my birthday over a year before, had come. I was at the end. I stayed, and, at last, the doctor opened the door.

That cold and rainy morning, as the door opened, I began a passage slow and stormy and not yet over. It was a journey of what, perhaps self-discovery and change? Robert Oppenheimer said once that atomic physics was only the second great interest of his life; his psychoanalysis was the first. I would not have understood what Oppenheimer meant, that January morning.

I began by explaining my problem to the doctor and setting forth what I wanted. Even with him, particularly with him, I could not let down my defenses. I said that my doctors had told me I was in depression with periods of acute anxiety. I said that the distress from this interfered with and, in one case, actually stopped my work and social life. I wanted relief from the symptoms. I wanted to restore my self-confidence so that I could pick up my career once again with the zest and motivation that I had brought to it in the past. I was 40, and over the years, I had built a reputation of integrity and intelligence in Washington and in the company where I worked. I had every expectation that over the next 20 years or so, my career would lead to responsible appointments in government and executive responsibilities within my company. The only obstacle to this was my depression with which I had wrestled unsuccessfully for a year and the reason I had come to seek help.

My presentation was calm and rational, although taut. My voice was gravelly. My hands shook and my body was tense. It was a humiliation for me to be in a psychiatrist's office. Throughout my life, I had handled my emotional problems without help. I had handled polio and the resultant severe paralysis with my own resources. I had constructed a life of notable success. The fact that I was there in his office that rainy morning was a major admission that something beyond my control had gone wrong. I did not like that one bit. I was acutely uncomfortable.

The doctor was nice enough. He was *quiet*; he moved *quietly* without quick or wasted motion as though he had planned to light his pipe *so*, as though he planned to cross his leg *so*. His voice had that measured, balanced, creepy quality psychiatrists seem to affect. He had a beard and a pipe, but I was pleased to see that he had no couch. He was very calm as though there was time enough to spare.

The man was roughly my age. Gauging from the books in his bookcase, we shared some interests. The furnishings in the room were puzzling. There were some nice pieces, but they did not fit together. They said nothing consistent about the room's owner. A motel room has a bland, meaningless consistence. This small room was anything but bland. Strong forces were at work here, but nothing in this room let on what they were. The only thing I remember about the man's clothes is that he wore no necktie, as though he were rather determined about wearing no necktie.

He did not really say anything. I told him what was wrong and what was to be put right. He asked a question or two, here and there, nothing out of the ordinary. At the end of the hour, he asked whether I thought I could work with him, and I replied I supposed so. He said he thought he could work with me. He suggested we find an hour suitable to our schedules and meet again next week. And that was it.

What a strange way to make a living. What a lot of money he charged to sit, listen, and puff a pipe. Nevertheless, he did seem to understand what I described and take it seriously. This, in retrospect, was important. What was happening to my life was deadly serious. No one I had talked to, not friend nor loved one, could be made to understand the dreadful nature of my despair or my inability to handle it. In fact, they denied it. They said to forget it, that it does not exist. I knew it did, and their denial of what I knew was real made me feel crazy, depressed and crazy. I was so alone. The doctor did seem to understand. Furthermore, he did not draw back—as my friends appeared to do—from the horror at work in my head. It was a cold comfort, but a real one I took away with me that morning. My visit to the doctor was admission that I could not continue by myself. I had come to ask for help, and that in itself was a beginning. I had held out my hand, and it had been grasped. That in itself was hope.

We met twice a week in the dark winter mornings before my work-day. The mornings grew light as winter became spring, spring became summer. Speaking with a seriousness I considered irrelevant, the doctor instructed that I should exercise, eat well, and get plenty of sleep. As I had struggled with insomnia over the last several years, he prescribed sleeping pills to help me reestablish my sleep patterns. What seemed a rather maternal concern with my rest and well-being turned out to be very practical advice. The emotional turmoil I experienced over the course of my treatment was physically exhausting and required all the strength I could summon.

Nothing much seemed to be happening. True, I had gone to the doctor because I feared the return of major depression, and this had not occurred. I was depressed, sometimes deeply so, but never as I had been the year before. The sessions were helpful in devising strategies for coping with the dinners and the trips, which had become so difficult. Such strategies were at best stopgap measures. They bought time, but resolved nothing.

After some six months, the doctor pointed out that I was no longer acutely depressed. And that was so. "You are free to go," he said. "Or," he said, "you can begin psychoanalysis and see if you can determine what has caused your depression. See if you can change it." And so, I began my analysis, meeting with the doctor four times a week.

I quit my job and retreated into my small house in the woods. I had a publlisher's contract to write a biography of President Herbert Hoover and I began to work on it.

The next several years of analysis required a courage beyond anything I had believed myself capable. There were to be periods of extreme danger to myself, perhaps even to others. The dictionary defines psychoanalysis as a process based on the theory that ". . . abnormal mental reactions are due to repression of desires consciously rejected but subconsciously persistent." I was to find myself to be a person of strong, even violent passions, severely and harshly repressed.

As the analysis progressed, and as my long-suppressed desires appeared, the fear with which I fought their appearance grew to panic. The torture of years of self-denial caused a fury beyond my power to control. The danger of suicide and violence was something I lived with for many, many months.

For example, in the spring of my second year in analysis, I began, in reluctant and halting fashion, to talk about my relations with my mother. I was smooth, almost glib, in describing her curious, cool way of mothering. Gradually, I became less glib as I plowed more deeply into my feelings and memories. I was not accustomed to strong feelings; in fact, they terrified me. In a real and physical manner, feelings terrified me. As it turned out, they had always frightened my mother. From infancy, I had repressed my strong feelings about mother. Now, after 40 years of repression, they were coming to the surface into my conscious thoughts.

Very strong feelings, indeed, were being aroused by this talk of mother causing a massive conflict. I was going crazy trying to repress the thoughts, while at the same time in analysis, I was trying to recover them from the past. I was at war with myself. At one point, absolutely in panic at what I was attempting, I called my doctor on a Sunday and blurted out in hysterical voice that I could not be responsible for what we were trying to do, that it was very dangerous for him, as for me, and that he must be very careful. To this veiled threat, he made no reply other than to say that he would be careful.

I began to slip back into depression, and I seemed powerless to stop the slide. This return to depression made me frantic. During my mornings, I was at work on my biography of Herbert Hoover. Always before, my reaction to depression had been to work hard, to work harder, to lose myself in my work. This is the path I had tried so painfully during my major depression of the year before. Curiously, it had been Hoover's strategy, too. During the Great Depression with the collapse of his administration and reputation, Hoover himself became chronically depressed. Hoover worked through the night, daily, month after month, trying to break his depression. He was no more successful at it than I had been. But now, I sought relief in my Hoover book; I sought strength and protection from Hoover. He had lived through his depression; I would live through mine.

Work would carry me through, I thought. I was wrong—not this time. Never again would I be able to suppress my feelings by drowning them in depression and then working my way out of the depression. I did not know this, though, and I worked with a madman's intensity on the project, but nothing went right. I cannot write without confidence, and I had no confidence left. My work was in shambles.

One day, the doctor told me what I already knew. "You are in depression," he said, "and we cannot do analysis when the patient is in a depressed state." He prescribed increasing doses of an antidepressant drug. Persuaded, perhaps, by my assurance in the way I talked to him of my mother, he could find no psychological reason for my depression. He believed at the time, that it might be organic in nature. The antidepressant would stimulate the secretion of some gland in my brain, and the secretion would blow away my depression.

The pills were tiny, orange with black dots. I was quite hysterical with fear by now. I soon developed side effects—virtually every single side effect listed in the pharmacopoeia. I was dreadfully doped. I lost my sense of balance. Getting up in the morning was a terrible agony. I sat through the day, staring at my books and papers, unable to work. The depression had clamped down upon me like a steel trap. It was all as it had been before, but now I was in the grip of a fearful drug as well. Soon, I lost control of my anal and urinary sphincters. This development was most frightening of all, reminding me of my period of agony and helplessness at the onset of polio when I was totally paralyzed, encased in an iron lung.

The climax came quickly. Unable to work, unable so much as to read the paper, I called my mother, asking her to come and sit with me to help my passage through the day. This, too, was a throwback to polio days when she had sat in a straight-back chair beside the iron lung as I struggled with the disease. I wanted her beside me again.

Mother said she would come, but she had an errand or so to do on the way over. She arrived over an hour late. She made some coffee and sat across the room from me, smoking a cigarette, thumbing through the pages of a *New Yorker*. Her presence, late or not, was sufficiently relaxing that I was able to make it to the bathroom for my first bowel movement in two days. Upon my return, I told her about my anal sphincter and my fears about my bowels. I had never, during polio, my rectal impaction, or since that time, spoken to her on the subject. She looked up from her magazine and laughed: "*Never* worry about bowels," she laughed, "never *worry* about that."

I think, in retrospect, it was then I was first aware, first felt that I wanted to *kill her*. I said nothing, in no way gave myself away, but that was when I felt it. My mother was so far removed from my life as a cripple, from my emotional life, so unaware of what I felt that she could say, "Don't worry about that." I was dumbfounded. My fury was murderous. In one blinding moment, I understood why I had spent a lifetime in denial: my mother was a stranger, and she had always been a stranger to my needs.

Like a stranger, she got up to go; she had shopping to do. If I wanted to come to dinner, she warned, remember that Father insisted upon starting drinks at six, so be on time. And then, she was gone, leaving me to my dark and loathsome fears—made more fearful yet by my discovery of my feelings toward her. Helpless and abandoned by my mother *one more time*. Quite literally, I could *not* bear it.

I did go to dinner with my parents. I drove very slowly because of the difficulty I had controlling the car. In their living room, I sat in the barrel chair, rather than on the couch, because it was easier to transfer to the chair from my wheelchair in my dopey state.

Father brought me a drink. I leaned to pick it up from the end table. Mother said something. I do not know exactly what, and I would like very much to know. As she spoke, the great taboo feeling, my hate and my desire to kill her, sprang forth in me. Simultaneously, sprang forth my determination to suppress this feeling at whatever cost, including my own death. At this moment of explosive, impossible conflict, I pitched forward onto the floor into convulsions.

I regained consciousness in the emergency room of the hospital. I was very sleepy, but very content. I asked my parents to take me to their home and put me to bed. I never wanted to live alone again, I said. I wanted to come home. In fact, I had amnesia and could remember nothing.

My memory returned over the next several days, although my depression did not. It was gone. I stayed several months with my parents, while I continued analysis. I could not remember for many months the subject on which we had been working in analysis. Gradually, I edged back inevitably to the all-important basis of my emotional life—my relations with my mother. At last, I recalled the cause of the depression, the convulsions, and the amnesia. Gradually, with difficulty and pain, I was able to resurrect and reconstruct and trace out the development of my life with mother. Slowly, I came to know the causes, the origins, the layer upon layer of misunderstanding. Slowly, I came to some sort of terms with the dreadful destructive fury I had found within myself, and I learned to accept it without fear. Freud never promised happiness, but he did talk of peace and relief.

Gradually, and I only became aware of this much later, my fear of the psychiatrist began to ebb away. I came to trust his restraint, his reserve. He was particularly careful to display no opinion, emotion, or expression whatsoever, sometimes holding himself frozen, as, slowly, I began to work out before him the fears that had brought me to treatment. During certain severe and crucial sessions, he said nothing at all. When he did speak, it was to summarize or give structure or shape to what I had said or to reinforce conclusions I had reached. And always, always, he kept me focused and honest.

Whatever was going to happen was going to be the result of my own effort. Had the doctor led me and had I found my happiness under his direction, I would have been exchanging my unhappiness for a dependence on him. This would have been a dependence I did not want and he would not accept. There were sessions when my despair would have wrung tears from a rock. During suicidal episodes, the danger under which I worked must have aroused his considerable concern. If so, he never allowed it to be seen. These were important times and critical matters were under review. Interference from the doctor or anything other than consistent support could have broken my confidence in my ability to do what I was attempting or provide an escape from the wretched unpleasantness of the task. Either event would have been quite disastrous for me.

When first I set to work, I did not know what I was doing. I did not know how to "work," and the doctor was not telling me how. This procedure accounts for the rather aimless feeling of the first months. Slowly, I came to focus on a single subject, to worry it, and, slowly, to unfold it, its history, its meaning, its importance. At the core, this was what I was doing. My resistance to this process of self-discovery produced many detours, much anxiety, and it confused the focus of my work for weeks at a time. It is my nature to proceed by fits and starts, which, when they came, were sometimes both explosive and unexpected.

I developed what might be described as an erratic, circular process. After weeks of thrashing anxiety, I would lurch forward into extraordinary insight, which would invariably be followed by violent recoil. There were two things going on during all this time: recovery and discovery. Discovery certainly impeded recovery. Discovery reordered the dismantlement of my psychic defenses. Recovery required a bolstering of these very defenses. The discovery process, rather than curing my depression, served to enhance it. Thus, for a time, I was in the curious state of actively aggravating the condition that had driven me to the doctor in the first place.

To my disappointment, I found there would be no magic involved in our sessions. There was no mystery to the procedure. The process was simplicity itself: What was it that had caused me unhappiness throughout my life? What caused my uncertainty and my fear? Why did I react in such a manner to such a situation? Where had it started; how had it developed? What were the facts of my situation, and what was the product of my emotional development? Equipped with this knowledge of myself, what could I do to change what could be changed and to accept what could not?

That is all there was to it. Thousands and thousands of dollars, years of effort, and that is all there was to it.

As I worked, as I sorted out the various episodes of my life, looked at them for their emotional content and meaning, discerning their importance to me and, more importantly, my reaction to them, certain patterns began to emerge. Strains would reappear again and again: reaction to stress, feelings about myself and about others. Events triggered obsessions, obsessions triggered actions, actions triggered events; the same reactions over and over again. There was a pattern, a predictable, even comprehensible, pattern to all this.

My dawning understanding was sporadic and incomplete. What came to be my diagnosis can only be seen by me in retrospect. My thrashing about within the process and my thinking were too erratic to provide an orderly statement of what was wrong and what would be required to set it right.

A diagnosis *did* form, however. It was difficult to accept because it located profound problems within me so deeply and firmly lodged that I despaired. Even their discovery seemed at the very cost of my self-respect and my dignity, or what was left of it. I despaired of adjusting to these discoveries; altering or ending them seemed to be overwhelmingly impossible. It was a miserable time.

I persevered. I came to accept that, for whatever reasons, I was emotionally crippled. Throughout my life, I appeared cheerful but was unhappy. The appearance fooled family and friends and confused me badly. I was reluctant to give up the appearance for the fact, but it was necessary. I was a sensitive, intelligent person of strong passion severely repressed. The surprising passion terrified me, and I did not know how to end, nor did I wish to end, the repression with which I had throttled my passions throughout my life. The appearance and the repressions served to cloak certain facts:

I had never accepted my physical handicap. I despised my body and all its works. This attitude had been so, long before polio. After polio, I simply finished off the job of amputating my body and its needs from my intellect. Its needs simply did not exist. The body was slave to my will. There was no congress between mind and body, none.

So deeply did I despise my body, I searched for additional ways to burden and humiliate it. This is, of course, what masochism is about. The crisis, which had brought me first to the doctor, can be represented in these terms. The body had at last rebelled; the slave would take no more. At the height of this crisis, I had denied it all—rest, nourishment, care, and pleasure in some crazy wild-eyed effort to bring my body back under discipline. The inevitable breakdown, when it came, came both in body and mind.

It became apparent that my problem with my body and my handicap was only symptom of a larger, more difficult problem. I despised myself. Within me, a seething fury was bent on self-destruction. The passion I had repressed was out to kill me. The masochism I practiced on my body was but a part of the self-punishment. There were, of course, no body pleasures, but, in addition, I allowed myself no other pleasures. No matter how spectacular my achievements might be, there was no pleasure in them. Whatever my creative work might be, there was to be no pleasure. In some deep, profound despairing place, I was unworthy, and there was no hope for me.

Most ghastly of all, I had placed myself beyond human concourse. I was unworthy, like a leper in exile; I was an outsider. So awful was my inside, I could reveal it to no one. I deserved no love, no comfort, no affection, and I refused all. Because I was weak, I could show no weakness. Because I craved love, I could allow myself none. Others could be weak and find solace, but not I. Others fell in love, married, had children, matured, experienced all the ups and downs that living brings—the comforts and distractions of loving another—but not I.

Last, my performance, what the world saw of me, covered all. I pleased others, not myself. It was my job to please others. If they were pleased with me, I was pleased or thought I was. If they were displeased with me, I was wretched. I had given away control over my happiness to others. If these others walked away—as invariably they did in search of someone who could respond to their need for love and comfort, for human intercourse—they took with them all my hopes for self-respect.

I had lived my life on a surface that was without flaw. There could be no sign to others of what lay underneath. The performance was in no sense sustaining, and, yet, so conditioned was I, there was no way of giving it up. There was no honesty, no happiness, no peace.

I was trapped within my performance. I could see the world out there but it was as if I were seeing it behind a plate glass window. The window stood between me and life, between me and other people between me and my world. Now I had smashed the plate glass window. I was wounded by the flying glass. Now what?

It took a long time to come by this diagnosis, longer still to accept. It was a dreadful diagnosis, but it was honest. For the first time in my life, I had been honest.

Of course, the formulation of the diagnosis had been no orderly affair. My search to isolate the elements, my effort to determine what had caused these elements to develop, and my struggle to alter or accept what I had discovered—none of this was orderly. The process is subtle and specific, different with each element, interrelated to all other elements, and constantly changing within itself. The process resists generalization. You could say I was finding out what made me unhappy. I was discovering what caused my depression. I was giving intense and structured attention to my troubles, the kind of thoughtful attention I had always given to my job, but never to myself.

A diagnosis is not a cure. Identifying what is wrong will not make it right. Identification of the wrong, however, is a necessary step, an integral, essential part of the cure process. Isolation of a deep-seated fear, familiarization with it, careful and extensive discussion of the fear, tracking it back to its origin in one's past history—this process makes it common currency. Its shock value is gone. Talking about a fear makes it less fearful; the fear remains, but you learn to accept it and to live with it as part of your makeup. The tremendous effort to repress the fear, the anxiety caused by its denial are stilled. The need for repression and denial evaporates, and, sometimes, the freedom and release experienced is euphoric. Sometimes, the freedom takes longer to sense because it is hard to believe that a deep-seated horror, which has dogged you throughout a lifetime, has at last been met in its totality and stilled. A lingering belief persists that it will return as virulent as ever in a new guise, the same old horror. And so it will, over and over. For a moment, the same old anxiety will grip you, the same old feeling of helplessness and doom. This feeling will last, however, only as long as it takes to recognize the new disguise. Discovery will not take long, and with discovery will come a renewed confidence, a renewed sense of freedom.

So, after some two years of my program of extensive, intensive self-analysis, I was able at last to give thought to goals, to what I wanted to take from all this analysis. I had my diagnosis. What did I want to do with it? I knew what I was. What was it I wished to be? What could I make of it all?

After thought, I drew up a contract, which I presented to my psychiatrist. It set the direction I wanted my analysis to take and staked out the results I was after. I wanted the psychiatrist to understand the direction and results I was looking for. He called them reasonable and possible. At this point, our work and our relationship took a new turn.

Originally, I had resented the need for a psychiatrist and feared working with him. He seemed to hold frightening, if mysterious, powers over me. During the long months of crisis, he had seemed a stern master, remote yet steady. Now he was becoming a partner in the reconstruction of my life, in the process of my growth into emotional maturity. It was not that he, his pipe, his living room had changed; it was that my perception of him—and of myself—had altered.

A consumer's group has studied psychotherapy from the patient's viewpoint, that is how to get the most for your money. The study recommends shopping around and discussing with the therapist the purpose of the projected therapy, the results expected, and the time required to obtain such results. The study suggests drawing up a contract of agreement between patient and therapist, containing purpose, time, and costs of treatment. Perhaps this advice is of value to the patient suffering premature ejaculation or persistent acne. This advice is of no value; it is irrelevant and even pernicious when applied to my experience. When I began analysis, I was on a breakdown course. My idea of what had gone wrong and what was necessary to put it right was itself the product of a mind that was not well. I could not see the facts of my situation, nor could I stand to feel the emotions at work within me. Any diagnosis, any contract I might have drawn up, would have been no more than a product of my disorder. How could I know whether I could "work" with the doctor when I had no idea what "work" meant and no idea as to where this work would take me. The only thing I could have done was what I did: start working blindly, trusting that my judgment of his ability and character was accurate and that we could understand each other. As it turned out, we could. In those early days, I was playing for keeps, and the risks were total; therapy would work or it would not. I could see no second chance. I allowed myself no alternative.

The personal progress toward understanding and direction, therefore, had been substantial. The contract was "reasonable and possible." And a new life began.

HOBART WILSON

Hobart Wilson is a sort of hero of mine. He had the guts to act out the anger I was feeling so intensely in the 1970s. Hobart came into my life in 1987. I am sorry I never got to meet him. I only learned about him from a newspaper account after his death.

The story stayed with me. I was so interested in the man that I went to the courthouse and read the transcripts of his trials. I tried to reach his family but could not do so. I did have a long informative discussion about Hobart with the judge he called a son of a bitch.

Hobart had a tough hand to play in the game of life, yet he played it with a certain kind of class and bravado. And when he could not take it any more, he killed himself and took out an innocent able-bodied person in the process.

I think most disabled people have an aspect of Hobart in their character. I know I do. I understand the anger, the frustration, the "born to lose" self-doubt just beneath the surface. No wonder Hobart said, "Damn the world." I say it sometimes, too. This piece has not been published before.

HOBART WILSON was a street punk, the worst. He was a greaser; he talked dirty, and he never fought fair. He lived hard and died young. His life was not much different from that of the others caught up in the urban jungle. Not much different except for one thing—Hobart was a paraplegic.

How does a paraplegic adjust to his condition? The adjustment is not easy, and there are not many role models to choose from. Some adopt the part of the chronic patient. They become the object of the ministrations of the doctors and the nurses and the therapists, taking their medicines, doing their exercises, active participants in the medical model of disability. Others choose to play the part of "super crip." They accept a lifelong competition with the fit. They are out to prove that not only are they equal to the nondisabled, they are better. They will outperform; they will out-achieve, work longer, rest less, even be healthier than the able-bodied. Their hero, the champion "super crip," was, of course, Franklin D. Roosevelt. Hobart Wilson, Jr., chose neither of these paths. He pioneered a third.

Junior, as he was called by his family, was born March 12, 1955, in Pineville, Kentucky. He was the youngest of four sons, and he was named after his father, who died when the boy was young. The father was buried, where he had lived, in the hills of Harlan County. The Wilsons were mountain folks—proud, independent people—typical of the county made famous by the Hatfield-McCoy feud.

When Junior was three, the family moved to Montgomery County, Maryland, a suburban region just outside of Washington. The little boy loved cars and mechanical vehicles of all kinds. He would play on them; at the age of five, he fell off a tractor, breaking his spine, paralyzing the lower half of his body forever. Because of internal injuries and complications, the doctors at first did not expect Junior to survive for long. His mother said, "After the accident, they told me he wouldn't live a year." Junior fooled the doctors. He had a lot of love from that close, proud family. As his mother told a reporter once, "He was the baby. He always got what he wanted. If he said, 'Let's have lemon pie tonight,' why, there would be a lemon pie." Junior survived, but he was in and out of the hospital for the rest of his life. He was upon occasion very sick with infections and kidney stones. He had not been expected to live but a year, his mother mused, ". . . but with the help of the Lord, he lived 21."

Junior's legs never grew much longer. As an adult, he was just five feet tall, had he been able to stand. Even though his shoulders and biceps were well developed, he never weighed much more than 90 pounds.

Junior never used a wheelchair, nor did he bother with braces and things. He rode about on a skateboard-like device of his own making. This was a piece of plywood about four feet long with a layer of foam rubber and a fabric cover. For wheels, he used wheels taken from a grocery cart. These do not work well at best, on occasion they jam and do not work at all. Junior was never far from his can of STP. Because his legs were small, skinny things, he was able to sit on the board with his legs crossed in a lotus position. Often, he would lean forward on his elbows, assuming a sphinx-like attitude.

Junior propelled himself by leaning forward, bringing the trunk of his body close to the surface of the board, and using his powerful arms, palms open against the pavement, to push forward, scooting across streets at an alarming speed. He could bounce himself up and down curbs. With the strength of his arms, he could pull his wasted body upstairs, bouncing step-by-step. In this fashion, he could go where he wanted when he wanted. Junior never cared much about traffic lights or crosswalks, and he would as soon wheel under a truck as around it.

For the years before his death at 26, Junior on his skateboard became a well-known figure in the Rockville area at the drag races, in the bars, and on the streets. He had a natural bent for mechanics and held jobs from time-to-time working on cars. He loved them and won trophies racing them. He was always buying, selling, fixing, and trading cars. His nephew estimates that Hobart owned between 35 and 40 cars during his short life.

Although Hobart worked upon occasion, he never did for long. He spent a good portion of his adult life in hospitals and a larger portion in jails. Hobart knew the prison guards well, just as they knew him. To this day, one of the Detention Center officials still keeps a can of STP in his drawer as a reminder of his paraplegic prisoner. Hobart Jr., was in and out of the police station so often that the department built a ramp for him. It is still referred to as the Hobart Wilson Memorial Ramp.

He was in court repeatedly, sometimes having two and three trials running concurrently. His court records fill many folders over several years. His career was known to every law enforcement officer in the county. One of them said to reporter Chip Brown of *The Washington Post*, as he was researching a story, "Hobart Wilson? Do you always write about garbage?"

Hobart never cooperated much with the police—or anyone else, for that matter—and his arrest records, of which there are a great many, reflect the frustration of the arresting officer. For example, one read:

> *Weight—?*
> *Height—?*
> *Hair—dark brown*
> *Eyes—brown*
> *Complexion—dark*
> *Date of birth—?*
> *Note—Suspect rides on platform and has no use of lower extremities.*

Hobart's criminal record is a long one. He was involved in several robberies. The tracks of his wheeled platform were found in the alley-way behind a store that had been burglarized. He was also convicted of such things as possession of a deadly weapon, drunk driving, trespass, breaking and entering, maiming, malicious destruction of property, and resisting arrest. He was what is called an unsavory character.

Junior carried an "Old Timer" switchblade knife, and he knew how to use it. This is how he would fight: He would try to knock his opponent down by charging at his ankles with his skateboard. Once his opponent was down at Junior's level, Junior would jump him. He stabbed and was stabbed many a time—once requiring 20 stitches to close the wound. The apparition of a wild man, seated on a skateboard, wielding a knife, caused a lot of people to keep their distance.

The general reaction to Hobart was a strong one. People are used to seeing the handicapped person as an object—an object of pity if he cannot "make" it, an object of admiration if he can. Hobart did not fit this pattern. He was nothing to admire, and, in his case, pity quickly turned to fear. The handicapped are used to hiding their feelings, keeping the unpleasant parts to themselves. Hobart let them all hang out—he let his anger show—and people called it garbage.

A typical case involved the charges of the man who lived next door to Hobart's widowed mother. According to Hobart, the neighbor had been insulting and harassing her over some matter. In response, Hobart threatened, as the neighbor reported to the court, ". . . to beat my ass."

The neighbor further testified that Hobart slashed four new Michelin tires and then threatened to kill him. Said the neighbor, "At which time he rolled toward me, raising his arm in a threatening manner." In this case, the court sentenced Hobart to a year in prison.

Hobart married a girl named Vickie, who cared deeply for him. After his death, she told reporter Chip Brown, "I don't think Junior was treated fairly. Nobody disliked him but police and judges. I know he wasn't all good. I know he had a high temper and a grudge against the world, but how would you feel if you were him and you heard people making smirky remarks?" As for his attitude toward his handicap, she said, "He never complained. I never heard him say, 'I wish it could be different.' He thought that's the way it was, that's the way it is, that's the way it's going to be."

The couple adopted a baby boy, and Hobart proudly named him Hobart Wilson III. They called him, "June Bug." Junior had tattoos on his biceps. As reporter Brown recalled, "His whole life was on his arms." There was a rose tattoo inscribed with his wife's name, Vickie. There was a complex pattern interweaving the names of his father, Hobart I, and his son, Hobart III, and, almost inevitably, for himself were the words tattooed, "Born to lose."

Vickie might have been right about Junior's never complaining; but he *was* angry—angry at himself and at others. One time in jail, in protest, he placed his leg between the bars and broke it like a matchstick in order to be transferred to the infirmary. In a curious choice of words, the officials called this a "tantrum."

At the end of his life, Hobart, who had the skill of a race car driver, took his hand-controlled car out on the highway. He revved it up to over 100 miles an hour, crossed the median line, and crashed head-on into an approaching vehicle. Junior was killed in the crash and fire that followed, and so was the innocent stranger driving the other car. The death of that stranger was accidental and unfair—just like Junior's paraplegia.

A feature story by Chip Brown in *The Washington Post*, June 15, 1981, about the life and violent death of Hobart Wilson produced a host of outraged letters. "Well, you people at the *Post* have sunk to an all-time low," said one. "I think it is about time we stop the sickening sympathy for those who deliberately break the law . . ." said another. The most moving and difficult letter came from the widow of the man who had been killed by Hobart's car. Said she,

> "So he was a cripple and a poor man; he should not have been driving in the first place. The story was written so that readers would feel sorry for a man who didn't deserve it, who felt sorry for himself and wanted to kill himself and didn't care who he took with him. Unfortunately, it was my good husband, the father to our two children."

The Wilson family put what was left of that small body into a coffin and loaded it onto the back of a pickup truck. They took it back home and buried Hobart beside his father in the hills of Harlan County, Kentucky. When reporter Brown interviewed Vickie upon her return from the burial, he says she said something that to this day makes his blood run cold when he thinks of it. She said, "I think he should have one decent thing said about him. If any of the high society took the time to talk to him, they'd see what a kind person he was. But they always had to be smart to him. Well, they can say what they want now. He is by his father where won't nobody push him no more."

It has been held as part of the crippled liberation movement that the handicapped person, if he is to be free, must have the right not only to compete and to succeed, but also to drop out, to fail. It may well be that by disposition and background, Hobart would have been a punk rebel, even had there been no accident. After the fall that left him a paraplegic, with defiance, he led his life as it had been dealt. Montgomery County, where Hobart lived, is a wealthy one, and it has all the latest rehabilitation services. But Hobart Wilson was not born to be rehabilitated. He was born to lose, and that's what he chose to do.

However, appraising his life as a paraplegic, he was no failure:

First of all, he escaped out of the medical model. Although his body was beset with ills and infections, he never became beholden to the doctors and nurses, the therapists and social workers.

Second, although paralyzed as an infant and raised by his mother in the confines of the family, he was able in due course to "separate" psychologically from her. As an adult, he proceeded to marry and have a family.

Third, he lived a life as independent as any man, making his own skateboards, cooking his own dinner on a hotplate on the floor. He had the full range of emotions from love to hate, and he was not afraid to express them.

These are important achievements for anyone. They are particularly difficult for the paraplegic to achieve. Once, in court, Hobart had an exchange with Judge Philip M. Fairbanks, which by now has become legendary in the Montgomery County courthouse. According to the transcript, Judge Fairbanks had just sentenced Wilson to three-and-a-half years in jail. Said Fairbanks: "I am not going to change my mind. . . . Mr. Wilson has been a problem, and he is just going . . ."

> Hobart: "Can I say something now?"
> Fairbanks: "You can say anything you want."
> Hobart: "You're a common son of a bitch."

The judge might have been common, but there was nothing common about Hobart. He was one of a kind.

GREGOR,
THE COCKROACH

This is an allegory of sorts, a shameless steal from Franz Kafka's "Metamorphosis".[1] It has not been published before.

GREGOR AWOKE WITH A START as the alarm sounded. The early morning sun streamed across his bed. Shutting his eyes to the light for a few more moments of sleep, Gregor tried to turn over.

Somehow he was stuck. Flat on his back, he could not turn over. Gregor looked down at his body and was startled to find that he had turned into a cockroach, a six-foot-long cockroach. "My God," he said. But all that came out were dry clicking sounds.

Gregor examined his new body. His eyes seemed to be mounted upon two flexible protuberances from his head which made it easy to see in all directions. His head merged as one piece into the trunk of his body which was now a long cigar-shaped tank. This tank or shell

---

[1]Franz Kafka, "The Metamorphosis," trans. A.L. Lloyd (New York, W.W. Norton,1960)

seemed to be made of something like celluloid, perhaps cartilage. He had the sense that it was fragile. Along the length of this extraordinary new body of his, there emerged pairs of little arms, or maybe they were legs.

Gregor did not know why he had turned into a cockroach. It was very strange. He felt the same, he thought the same things, he was the same Gregor he ever was, except that here he was trapped in this bizarre body.

After some experimenting, he found that by waving his little arms and legs in the air *so*, and by rolling from side to side *so*, he could roll over onto his stomach. And then, using his arms and legs he was able to back straight off the end of the bed, slowly, slowly, until gravity would tilt his body downward and it touched the floor.

He was trotting into the kitchen when his mother saw him and screamed. He tried to reassure her: "It's me, Gregor, your son."—but this came out as a series of dry clicks and it did little to calm the poor woman. His father already had gone to work.

That night they had a family meeting. Normally these meetings were held around the dining room table, but in this case they had it on the kitchen floor. Given the circumstances, it seemed the best that could be done. Gregor didn't like seeing his mother sitting cross-legged on the floor—she looked uncomfortable. He tried to reach out to her with one of his little arms, but she moved away.

Dr. Kollesard was at the meeting. He had been the family doctor for many years. Normally, he did not make house calls, but in this case he made an exception. Kollesard had given Gregor a careful physical examination, admittedly a difficult business. The doctor found that Gregor had a pulse and a heartbeat, but they were much quicker than those of an ordinary human being. So too, his respiration was regular but different. He had no blood although there was a nicotine-colored fluid that the doctor was able to draw out. He said he would send it to the laboratory for a full analysis.

Kollesard tried to reassure the family, "It could be worse," he said. "Your son is in good health for a cockroach, as far as I can tell."

This did not soothe the distraught mother. "I don't want a cockroach for a son," she said. "Of course I love him, but what will the neighbors think?"

According to Dr. Kollesard who had a run a search on the medical computer system, Medline, there was no case in the literature similar to Gregor's. There had been a man in Minnesota who believed he had turned into a cow, but there had been no obvious bovine physiological changes to support the belief. When Kollesard did a Medline search for the word "cockroach," he drew a blank.

"The mind-body connection is a powerful thing," said Kollesard in a thoughtful way, putting his fingers carefully together. He indicated that perhaps some sort of obscure, yet intense, psychosomatic stress reaction could be at the root of Gregor's transformation into a cockroach. "I suggest a full evaluation by a specialist in physical medicine and rehabilitation."

That night, Gregor's father rigged a ramp at the foot of the bed, using a piece of plywood from the garage. Gregor was able to creep up the ramp into bed under his own power. He lay in the dark, waiting for sleep. "Maybe when I wake up in the morning, all this will prove to have been a dream."

When he woke up the next morning, he found he was still a cockroach. Using the plywood ramp again, Gregor was able to climb up and into the back hatch door of the family station wagon for the ride to the rehabilitation clinic. He was not very comfortable; he was afraid that his outer shell would bruise on the rough carpeting. It was good however to be out, even reassuring to see people out on the streets going about their ordinary affairs.

Dr. Ransard was a fat man with thick lens eye-glasses. "Don't worry," he told Gregor's mother. "I will soon have your boy back upright on his own two feet—er, two of his feet."

When his mother looked uncertain, Ransard continued, "It is a matter of proper orthotic prostheses—braces—and careful muscle reeducation. We will map out a program of physical therapy sessions, over the course of which we will develop the muscles of Gregor's last pair of legs and stretch them, so that properly braced, they will support the weight of his upright body.

"With the assistance of computer programming—and we *are* very up-to-date at the Ransard clinic—heh, heh—we will soon have your son's braced legs moving forward, first one and then the other. Just like walking." Ransard positively beamed.

"It is my expectation that, over time, Gregor's braced legs will develop muscle mass and grow in stature while his other arms and legs, or whatever, will atrophy into useless appendages. A plastic surgeon could then remove them with minimal trauma."

They started physical therapy the next day. It was a painful business: exercising his back legs did not hurt but the stretching did. His legs had a more than right angle bend at the joint and the business of stretching them out straight was agony. "Clickety, clickety, clickety click," Gregor would gasp, waving his little arms in the air.

"Do you think he's feeling pain?" his therapist Doris would ask the other therapists. They could not decide.

After two months of this, the looked-for day came when Gregor was to stand erect for the first time. His mother, who usually did not stay around for the therapy session, was there as was his father who had taken the afternoon off from work.

The little braces were affixed to his rear legs and straightened and locked. The pain was intense but Gregor was proud that this much had been achieved. A parachute harness was—rather cleverly—attached to his body. This the doctor had suspended from the ceiling by a block-and-tackle arrangement.

When all was ready, Gregor's body was gradually raised to an erect position. At first most of his not inconsiderable weight was supported by the harness; his feet were just brushing the floor. But with both Doris and his father steadying his body and with the doctor working the ropes of the harness, slowly Gregor's entire weight was lowered onto his legs.

Gregor was excited to be upright. The harness went slack; Doris and his father relaxed their grip. Gregor was standing! He felt terribly dizzy; all at once, he was very close to blacking out: he thought that gravity must be pulling all the fluids from his head. He slumped forward, twisted, and as he did so, there was a loud pop. His right leg snapped off, severed at the place where it joined the trunk of his body. The juncture was a knoblike thing, and the leg just popped out of it. It made a terrible sound. Gregor never forgot that sound.

There was no wound, no blood, nothing. Nothing but the poor little lifeless leg with its peculiar little aluminum brace attached to it. Dr. Ransard later threw both away in the trash.

The next day, when it was time to go to physical therapy, Gregor hid under his bed and refused to come out when his mother asked him. That night, there was another family meeting on the kitchen floor. His mother and father decided that Dr. Ransard's approach to the problem was perhaps not working very well.

Ransard wanted to arrange things—braces, harnesses, and such— so that Gregor *looked* normal. That was no cure. Gregor's mother put the finger on the problem. "Even if he is standing up, he is still just a big cockroach. What's the future in that?" So Gregor stopped going to the Ransard clinic.

After stopping physical therapy, Gregor became very inactive. "Just a big cockroach," he remembered his mother had said and she was right. He refused to go out of the house, even for drives. Most afternoons he spent in his room, lying on his bed watching Oprah.

At the request of the family, Dr. Kollasard talked to the physician who had treated the man in Minnesota who thought he was a cow. The physician reported the man had made remarkable progress through psychoanalysis, intensive and extensive. He no longer thought of himself a cow except on occasions of extreme stress; he was married, the father of a baby girl and currently working as a shoe salesman.

The family went together to meet with the analyst who had been recommended. His name was Herschel Brattle and he was a little man, not much more than 5 feet tall, very intense, with a precise little military mustache. "Yes," he said, fiddling with his pipe as he spoke, "Yes, the mind is capable of extraordinary things. Certainly." He paused, "A person can be so terrified of taking a misstep that he cannot take a step at all—and this we call hysterical paralysis. A person can become so bound up by the strictures he imposes upon himself that he becomes as immobile as a statue—and this we call catatonia."

Brattle was silent for quite a while. Gregor had been dragged up on the doctor's chaise lounge by his father and Dr. Brattle. Gregor crouched there rather awkwardly on his arms and legs. Staring intently at the large cockroach before him, the analyst continued, "In the present case, we have, it seems, an extreme case of—uh—an *id* so battered and defensive as the result of such severe, if at present unknown trauma, as to actually have constructed for the body a full-length shield.

"If—and this is of course all important—*if* the patient is willing to make an absolute commitment to the analysis, it should be possible to peel away the protective layers and uncover the cause of his terrible trauma. And then as the patient confronts his trauma and comes to terms with it, his body will no longer need to encase itself in the armor of a cockroach. Your son will then be cured!"

Analysis with Dr. Brattle was very expensive. Gregor's mother had to go back to work to help pay for it. Every weekday, Gregor was dragged up on Dr. Brattle's couch. The 50-minute analytic session was trying. Brattle was a strict Freudian and said very little. Gregor would go over in his mind, over and over, the events of his life, looking for clues to his condition. At first he tried to convey something of his thoughts to Brattle, but all he could manage was a series of clicking sounds. Brattle, who busied himself working on a large needlepoint rug, soon came to pay little attention to his patient.

After several months of this, Gregor put his little foot down. It made no sense for his parents to be spending their life's savings for him to lie on a couch watching Dr. Brattle make a rug. Besides, every time his mother looked at him, her eyes would cloud over with unhappiness. He did not like being the cause of such continuing pain—to say nothing of the expense. Gregor decided to run away.

He was tired of being hidden away in his back bedroom. Gregor knew his Mother didn't want the neighbors, the Jones, to see him in his present condition, but damn it. Maybe he was only a cockroach now, but he still loved the outdoors, the sunshine, and his independence. He had spent six months cooped up in the house with his parents—he was sick of it and he was sure they were too. It wasn't fair for them to have to struggle with what was, after all, his problem.

That night when the house was asleep, very carefully, Gregor backed down the ramp at the foot of the bed onto the floor. He tiptoed on his little feet to the window. It was a sliding panel opening to the patio. Slowly, for it was hard work, he inched the door open, first pushing with his hard snout, and then pulling with his first pair of legs. Gradually the door slid open; fortunately, the screen was not latched, and Gregor was able to slide it back. He scraped down the single step to the terrace and he was free. Across the lawn and down the alley, he hurried as fast as his little feet would carry him.

He was six blocks from the Weyland County Forest Preserve. If he could get that far without being seen, he was safe. The alley was dark, so that was all right. At the cross streets, he waited in the shadows until the coast was clear and then he scurried across.

He knew the woods well. He had grown up playing in them. There was a fallen tree trunk wedged up against a large boulder, maybe six feet across. Burrowing with his sets of legs, he shaped a trough in the ground beside the trunk under the rock. Gregor was all but hidden to passersby.

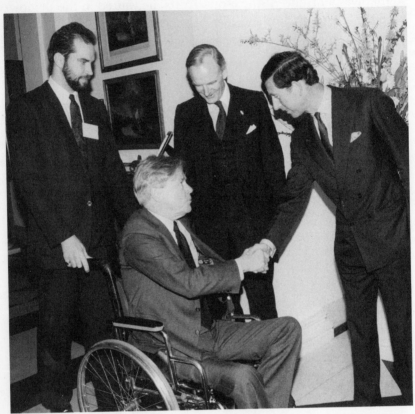

HRH Prince Charles is the honorary chairman of the Marshall Scholars Association. Here I am meeting him at the British Embassy. To the left is my nephew, Timothy L. Hermans and on the right, the British Ambassador, Sir John Ackburn.

THE THIRD SCORE YEARS

RENAISSANCE

THE 1980 WERE PRODUCTIVE years for the disability rights movement and they were productive years for me.

The Reagan and Bush years were tough. One after another of the programs protecting disability rights (accessibility compliance, mainstreaming, section 504) came under attack from conservatives in the Congress and the White House who were anxious to reduce the size and influence of the federal government. In each case, efforts to cut or end the program met with such an outcry from the disability community that they had to be dropped.

In the process, the disability community learned how to organize to protect their interests, how to use the media and, most importantly, how to make themselves felt in the halls of Congress. I believe the community also learned how to call upon the support of American society at large in their struggle for disability rights. In the 1980s, the "sleeping giant," as pollster Lou Harris called the tens of millions of disabled Americans, began to wake up.

Thus, ironically, at the end of a decade of attacks, the disability movement found itself stronger than ever before. It was this strength, the skill of the leaders of the movement, and the brilliant strategy of Evan Kemp, Boyden Gray and, yes, George Bush, that culminated in the passage in 1990 of the Americans with Disabilities Act. This unique bill of rights for disabled people is as important to the nation as the Civil Rights Act of 1964. It recognizes the full civil rights of disabled people and pledges the nation to support and enforce those rights. Such an acknowledgement and pledge have never been made before by any nation at any time. The world is a different place.

In the early 1980s, I was introduced to Evan Kemp. At the time, he was Director of the Nader-based Disability Rights Center. My first words to him were, "I understand you are a professional cripple. I don't like professional cripples." It is amazing he ever spoke to me again, but he did. We became—and remained—close friends.

I had been wrestling with my thoughts on disability. There was much I did not understand. So many emotions swirled around it: anger, fear, grief, and so many attitudes: ostracism, pity, paternalism. What *was* disability and why did it carry so much baggage with it? Evan and I began meeting weekly over dinner at a little restaurant called P Street Station. There we would talk and argue about disability. The more we talked, the more interested I became.

My writings of the 1980s and 1990s grew out of those talks with Evan. What, after all, is it to be disabled? Is it only a physical attribute or is it something that alters the whole person? Is it a bum leg or an entire culture with a unique way of looking at the world? These are the sorts of questions I pondered.

In working my way out of my depression, I had often compared myself with Franklin Roosevelt. He was a polio paraplegic and, as far as I knew, he had never experienced the psychological problems I was struggling with. He was OK but I was not. How come?

I decided to find out. It was 1982, the International Year of the Disabled. I applied for and received a fellowship from the Woodrow Wilson International Center for Scholars, which is housed in the Smithsonian Institution. The fellowship allowed me to research FDR through use of the vast resources of the Library of Congress. The book that resulted from my work at the Center, *FDR's Splendid*

Deception,[1] after 17 rejections, was at last published in 1985. A revised edition is still in print.

The rejections reflected, I believe, a certain puzzlement and discontent with the book's subject. The book was an analysis of the impact of paraplegia on FDR as a man and leader. It was not an "inspirational" book, nor was it a standard biography. It was not a medical book, nor a "how-to" live with your disability sort of thing. Book stores and libraries did not know where to shelve it. I remember I submitted a long excerpt for publication to the Center's distinguished journal, *Wilson Quarterly*. After a suitable period, its editor came to me to say that the article could not be printed in the *Quarterly*. He said the Quarterly was an intellectual and scholarly journal. Disability was not such a subject. Perhaps, he suggested, with a little reworking my piece might be accepted by one of those uplifting religious magazines passed out in Sunday schools! This was in the early 1980s when the idea that there were serious and, yes, intellectual issues surrounding the socialization of disability was unthinkable. The burgeoning field of disability studies had yet to be born.

The more I thought about disability, the more interested I became. In the spring of 1986, I decided to explore the social and moral aspects of disability. I was thinking of Simone de Beauvoir's *The Second Sex*[2] which is her exploration of what it is to be a woman in today's society. To find out, she searched through the various disciplines—history, anthropology, sociology, psychology, medicine, religion—compiling and analyzing what they say about woman. In my innocence, I thought I will write a book about my disability as Beauvoir wrote about her sex.

It turned out to be a lifetime project. The research is not easy. You cannot go to the card catalogue and look up, say, "ancient Greece, disability, attitudes toward." There is virtually nothing on disabled people in the library other than personal accounts and medical tracts. There has never been a book on the history of disabled peoples. Only now are people beginning to ask, "How is it that the disabled have been devalued, segregated, denied their civil rights for so long in so

---

[1] *FDR's Splendid Deception*, Vandamere Press, Arlington, VA 1994
[2] Simone de Beauvoir, *The Second Sex*, Random House, New York, 1990

many societies? Where did these ideas come from? What do they mean?"

The history of disability comes in bits and pieces. It lies in medical studies, diaries, letters, genre paintings, ceramics, Bible and religious studies. It hides in anthropological studies. Sometimes it is even found by its omission from a treatise.

Thanks to the support of the Director, Dr. Edmund Pellegrino, I became a visiting fellow at what is now the Center for Clinical Bioethics at Georgetown University. In my letter of application, I enclosed the following argument. In it I struggled to marshal my thoughts on what I hoped to do. I thought I could do it in a year. More than ten years later I am still at work.

THE ARGUMENT

The handicapped are a minority without a community. Isolated and uncertain throughout history, they have been largely without voice.

Into present times, the handicapped have been shunned, interned, and segregated. Into present times, they have been denied employment and education; their sexuality has been denied, and the Church has denied them the priesthood and forbidden them to marry.

The handicapped are members of society, and it is not surprising they share the values of their society. This means they have a *learned* inferiority; they have been taught dependency, denial, and low self-esteem. They have been taught to see themselves as chronic patients in a medical model—patients who never get well, rather than members of a minority in a civil rights model—citizens who must assert their rights or lose them.

This is a period of great ferment for the disabled. For the first time in recorded history, efforts are being made as a matter of public policy to integrate them into the mainstream of society. These efforts come at a time when there are a great many more handicapped persons than there ever before. Modern medicine is producing more chronically disabled people all the time. This is so because lives that hitherto were lost can now be saved, but at the price of permanent disability. Also, and for the first time, groups of the handicapped are now becoming politically active, publicizing and lobbying for their demands with a certain sophistication. Given the pattern of political awakening of other minority groups, it may happen the handicapped will come to have significant influence over the making of national policy in the years ahead.

These are events without precedence in the history of mankind. They attempt to reverse traditional attitudes and may even be seen to conflict with biological instinct for they are, in a sense, counter-evolutionary; they serve the preservation of the unfit. These events raise serious social and ethical issues for the disabled, for medicine, for the Church, and for society as a whole.

Such issues as these:

- Does the insistence upon saving and maintaining the life of the seriously disabled imply a societal obligation to ensure these survivors a certain quality of life?
- Can the quality of life become so burdened with disability as to render that life unacceptable? If so, when and by whom is it to be so judged; and after the judgement, what then?
- What light may the behavior and thought of other cultures shed on these issues? How may classical studies, economics, and philosophy be brought to bear? How may the handicapped themselves participate in the resolution of these issues?
- Doctors trained in the physiochemical theory of life are often unaware, or unwilling to become aware, of the major psychological aspects of chronic medicine. Treatments biologically helpful can be psychologically damaging. Thus, unwittingly, doctors often do great harm. How best may they be made aware of the harm they do?

- The handicapped fear, even hate, their doctors; for their part, doctors dislike their chronic patients. How may this shared hostility be overcome and communication improved?
- In rehabilitation theory, the handicapped are encouraged to expend the very limit of their emotional and physical strength necessary to hold down a job. Can such an expenditure be justified morally? Why is there so often a punitive quality to so much of rehabilitation?
- Medicine is obsessed with prosthetics for the disabled to make them *appear* what they are not. Is it not better to encourage the disabled to accept their diversity, rather than aid them in their denial of it?
- A third of the national's paraplegics live in chronic depression; suicide is their principal cause of death. Psychotherapy, although effective, is still virtually unavailable to a majority of these persons. Is this not an immoral state of affairs?

This was a stupendous project, and it turned out to be most difficult to research. I found out that disability in a social sense is not a subject that scholars study. For example: Very little, practically nothing, has been written about attitudes toward the disabled in ancient Greece. There is nothing on the portrayal of the disabled in 17th century Dutch genre art. The origin and practice of discrimination against the disabled by the major religions of the world have never been studied. The exclusion of disabled citizens from the civil rights protections of the U.S. Constitution has never been written about or analyzed.

I was overwhelmed by the size of my task and appalled by how difficult it was to ferret out even the simplest facts. Finally, I had to compromise. I wrote a book, *By Trust Betrayed*[3] about a particular episode in disability history. I wrote about the so-called "euthanasia" program of the Third Reich in which the physicians of Germany killed many

---

[3]*By Trust Betrayed: Patients, Physicians and the License to Kill in the Third Reich*, Vandamere Press, Arlington, VA, 1996

more than 200,000 of their disabled patients whom they judged to have "lives not worth living".

It seemed to me this catastrophe in our own times served to encapsulate and set forth in highly dramatic fashion many of the attitudes and prejudices that have dogged the life of disabled people throughout the centuries—and in today's America. It seemed to me the German physicians, with their mad efficiency and arrogant confidence in the infallibility of their judgment, did no more than act out in grotesque fashion the feelings toward the disabled that are widely shared, albeit unconsciously, by many in our society.

By the end of the decade, with the publication of my books and various articles and op-ed pieces, I found myself invited to address groups and organizations on issues of importance to the disability community. These speaking engagements made it necessary for me to travel back and forth across the country. I had not traveled, unless forced into it, since before my 1974 breakdown.

To travel again was difficult at first but over time it has become much easier. One reason is that travel *has* become easier for someone using a wheelchair. Airlines no longer blanch when you show up at the departure gate. Hotels know what you are talking about when you ask about door widths and numbers of steps. But the more important reason travel is easier is that I am better at accepting my neediness.

In the bad old days, I tried to be the "heroic" crip. I asked no one for help. I was determined to get into cars without help. I would transfer, all by myself, onto strange toilets even if the transfer was dangerous. I would lift myself into hotel beds even if the effort left me breathless and my muscles cramping. I insisted upon traveling alone; I even flew alone around the world. The tension and anxiety caused by this made travel a terror.

Now I no longer have the strength to pretend that I can live independently on the road. I need help with everything. If I am to travel, I now must travel with a helper. To my great surprise, this has made travel not only easier, but also fun. Over the years I have been fortunate to have had as helpers some excellent guys. They have been not only employees, they have become lifelong friends. They are Paul Waggaman, Frederick Alexander Sollock, Jeff Steinbach, Dan Virgilio,

J.P. Wirth and for the last several years, John Holstein. Thanks to their help, my life has become fuller and happier.

Now in the 1990s, I am in my sixties and I have used a wheelchair for more than 40 years. Thanks to advances in disability equipment, I use an electrically powered chair and drive a van with a remote-controlled electric ramp and powered hand controls. I can drive my van while seated in my wheelchair. These things give me an independence and range of movement greater than any I have had since I contracted polio in 1952.

In times past, I have been kicked out of movies, thrown off airplanes, and denied access to bars and restaurants. The Royal Academy of the Arts would not let me into its galleries because my chair was thought to be a hazard to serious art lovers who might trip over it. Providence Hospital here in Washington, for many years had not one bathroom that was wheelchair-accessible. Neither the Capitol nor the White House was accessible. When I worked for President Johnson, I had to urinate in a coffee can.

All this has changed. With the passage of the Americans with Disabilities Act, the nation is literally rebuilding itself to become accessible to the disabled. Public accommodations and transportation must make all reasonable efforts to provide access for the disabled. When I travel to a new place, I can usually count on accessible facilities for my use. This makes my life, and the lives of other disabled people much easier. This is why one sees so many more disabled people out in public places than ever before.

These physical changes are important. Even more important is what they symbolize. A curb cut is a curb cut, but it is also an invitation. It says to the disabled person, "Come out to the agora, come take part. You have as much right to participate in the affairs of society as anyone else. You are a welcome member!"

In recent years I have traveled the country speaking out on disability issues. As I see it there are two major matters facing our community, and they are interrelated: managed health care and assisted suicide. Neither managed care nor assisted suicide is, per se, necessarily a danger to disabled people if it is managed with an intelligence free of bias and a genuinely good and informed conscience. Alas, such intelligence and conscience are rare in the society of man.

The allocation of limited health care, by the very nature of the word "allocation," involves decision-making: who will receive the limited care and who will not. Such a decision contains an implicit "quality of life" judgement. In some way, patient A is more valuable, and thus more deserving, than patient B. Or as the Managing Director of the Partnership for Organ Donation said in announcing new criteria for whom shall receive liver transplants in the United States, "There's only so much room in the lifeboats, and a bunch of people are going to drown."

In a similar sense, questions on when to "pull the plug" in the terminal stages of life or when to assist in a self-administered suicide also involve morally weighted decision-making. Who is to make the decision that a patient's prognosis is hopeless? Who is so wise as to decide that my life or yours has lost its value? It's a tough call.

If history is an indicator, people with disabilities do not fare well when such decisions are made by people without disabilities. "I would hate to live like that," the able-bodied are apt to say. "I would rather be dead." It is because of such rationales, that few disabled people make it to the lifeboats.

I intend to say and to write more on such matters for as long as I am able.

FDR AND ME

Many disabled people have asked me if FDR should be a role model. This is my reply. I wrestled over this piece. It was only after I had carefully analyzed the impact that FDR hero worship had on my own life that I was able to see the damage I had done myself. FDR was a prisoner of his time and culture. Things have changed in our time and culture, and we disabled people are the better for it. This piece was originally presented as a speech in Anchorage, Alaska and later appeared in several disability newsletters.

I WAS A NEW DEAL CHILD. I was born within a month of Roosevelt's election in 1932, and for the first 13 years of my life, he was the only President there was. FDR could do no wrong in my eyes.

When FDR ran for his third term in 1940, I passed out campaign buttons. Four years later, I was a page at the Democratic Convention that nominated him President for the fourth time. In the floor demonstration, I carried a banner that read, "Don't Change Horses in Mid-Stream." That banner hung on my bedroom wall for years.

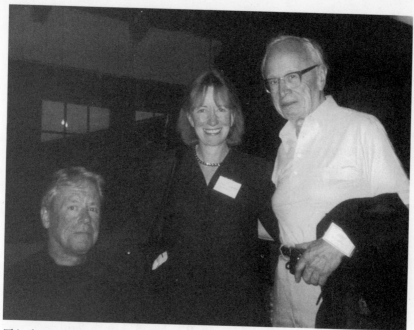

This photo was taken at Warm Springs, Georgia in April, 1995 on the occasion of the 50th anniversary of FDR's death. I am with fellow Roosevelt historians Doris Kearns Goodwin and Arthur Schlesinger, Jr.

Roosevelt entered my life again when I contracted a severe case of paralytic polio in 1952. After a year in hospital, I went to the Georgia Warm Springs Foundation for my rehabilitation. Roosevelt had created the Foundation in the 1920s and his ebullient spirit still pervaded the Foundation when I was there seven years after his death. FDR became my role model. He denied his disability and led a famously successful life.

Twenty years after Warm Springs, I found myself in deep depression. Clearly FDR's way was not working for me. It took all my energy to maintain my facade of success and confidence. There seemed to be nothing behind the facade.

I wondered about my hero, FDR. Had there been anything behind *his* facade? To answer this question, I began the research that resulted in my book, *FDR's Splendid Deception*, a psychological study of Roosevelt as a handicapped person.

This is what I found: FDR dealt with the fact of his paralysis by means of total denial. He never talked to anyone about the feelings generated by his loss, not to his wife, not to his mother, most probably not even to himself. Wife Eleanor is reported to have said, "You know he has never admitted he cannot walk." If someone was foolish enough to make reference to his disability, FDR would cut off the conversation with a cold fury.

I have known hundreds of paraplegics in my time, and for every single one, the fact of his paralysis is the central focusing event of his life. Surely, this was as true of FDR as it is of the others. FDR just refused to acknowledge or talk about the fact. This meant that a large part of his emotional life was off-limits. He shared his emotions with no one, and, thus, he allowed his handicap to isolate him from the comfort and support that love brings. This made him a remote and distant figure to his children. In part, it caused his wife to seek solace elsewhere. It also seems to have contributed to the mental and physical collapse of his secretary, who loved him dearly. The wreckage proceeding from FDR's closed mouth "courage" was everywhere.

I remember a rainy, cold November Sunday afternoon. I was out in my hand-controlled car at a Burger King. I was the only car in the parking lot, for every other soul in all of Washington was watching the Redskins. I was sitting in my car, working on one of the closing chapters of the book. It dealt with FDR's last year of life, when the strength of his remaining muscles began to fail. It was the very climax of World War II, and Roosevelt was carrying the heaviest leadership burden in the history of man. Burdened as he was, calling upon every last ounce of strength and energy his body could provide, his muscles failed him. This surely was a supreme betrayal, and, yet, he *never once* complained to anyone, so far as is known, about the loss of his muscle power, not even to his doctor, if that man's testimony is to be believed. His self-control was superhuman. He died before his time, lonely, depressed, and exhausted.

I, too, in recent years have experienced a serious loss of strength and endurance in my remaining muscle power. The doctors had assured me, just as they had assured FDR, that, once a polio-weakened muscle is retrained to strength, it will perform as any other muscle throughout the life of the patient. They were wrong, and today, this weakening is known popularly as post-polio syndrome. Whatever this loss of power is called, it has made me very angry, among other emotions.

It was there in that cold and rainy parking lot that I at last broke with the President of the United States. I would be goddamned if I would follow him, stiff upper lip, good soldier to the last. I would shout out my hurt to the skies, curse the fates, both mourn and celebrate my loss. FDR was a great man, a magnificent leader of world scale, but he was no longer my role model. He was Super Crip; I opted for human.

My feelings are mine; they go with the territory. People who love me will share these feelings, and, together, we will cope; more than that, we will prevail. This way lies survival. FDR's way leads to nowhere but a bleak isolation.

I have been going around the country promoting my book. In my talks to various groups, I try to explain my personal discovery/decision about FDR. As I do, I notice the handicapped people in the audience become very silent, very attentive. I think sometimes they hold their breath with the intensity of their silence—and their listening. There is then a long, maybe even *deep,* pause before they applaud. Afterwards, when they come up to me, they want to touch me. This has never happened to me before, but I think I know why. It is because they sense that I understand.

WHO CARES ABOUT
DISABLED PEOPLE?

I have been writing for publication my entire adult life, and I do not think any piece of mine aroused such fevered response as this one. The letters received by the editor were uniformly intelligent, but troubled.

I wrote the article as a disabled person—as a consumer, not a provider of medical services. I meant the article to be severely critical of the medical profession. My point was this: the incidence of mental illness among the disabled is high. The effectiveness of psychotherapy in the treatment of such illness is acknowledged. Yet, the disabled are widely denied the access to psychotherapy that is commonly available to "normals."

I see this as an accessibility problem. The handicapped have as much right of access to mental health therapy as they do to public transportation and post offices. The mental health professionals are avoiding treatment of the disabled, and will continue to do so until the disabled demand attention. An example of the current professional

Reprinted from *Social Policy*, Spring 1985.

attitude comes in a letter received by the editor from a rehabilitation psychologist. She found my article "boring." As an author I was stung by the comment, but as a paraplegic I was angered. The subject is boring only in the sense that continued television pictures of starving Ethiopians are boring. My fellow paraplegics are blowing their brains out because of untreated situational depression, and the professionals find this boring?

I feel strongly about this matter, and perhaps my feelings served to obfuscate my meaning. For example, a number of the handicapped who read the article seemed to think I was asking them to resign themselves to the obstacles of the present world, to give up the struggle for a barrier-free environment. I did not mean this at all.

I meant that we should not confuse the struggle for an accessible world with our need for emotional well-being. A handicap has emotional as well as physical components, and both must be acknowledged and tended. It is appealing and straightforward, but wrong, to say: if only we had kneeling buses and accessible subways, then our self-esteem would be restored.

In fact, something like the reverse is true. The better we feel about ourselves, the more healthy our self-esteem, the more effectively we can work to make the world accessible to all.

Sigmund Freud always found a good deal of antagonism toward his ideas and toward himself for advancing them. The response to my article indicates that this antagonism is alive and well.

THE MENTAL HEALTH of physically handicapped people—blind, deaf, and mobility-impaired persons—is a taboo subject. By and large, the problem is denied by the handicapped and ignored by psychiatry.

No one knows with fine accuracy how many, but there are over 30 million handicapped people in the United States. The development of various life-lengthening medical techniques means that there will be many millions more over the coming decades. No one knows with any accuracy the incidence of mental illness among handicapped people, but certainly it is not less than the incidence among the general population—and there are reasons to believe it is much greater.

Recently, a survey of available material on this subject was done for the National Institute of Mental Health by Richard H. Beinecke, himself a mental health therapist. The following facts are taken from Beinecke's study. They are sobering, indeed.

- Although for most categories of disability there are simply no figures on mental illness available, there are some reliable statistics for deafness. This is because of the research undertaken by Gallaudet College, a higher education institution in Washington, D.C., for the deaf. The medical model forces the handicapped person to repress as "unhealthy" the genuine feelings of anger, hurt, and grief at any substantial physical loss.
- There are some 13 million deaf and hearing-impaired persons of all ages in America. Hard of hearing children have been found some three to six times more likely to have emotional problems as they are growing up than do hearing children. The emotional health of deaf adults is the subject of controversy. They may or may not have a higher incidence of mental illness than do hearing people. But it is clear that the level of alcoholism and drug abuse is substantially higher.
- Yet, in all of America in 1976, there were only 20 psychiatrists working with deaf patients, and of these doctors only five had any knowledge of sign language. Not one of the doctors was deaf, and only 726 adult deaf persons received treatment.
- Also in 1976, only 16 psychologists (five of them deaf) worked with deaf patients, plus 27 psychiatric nurses, none of whom was deaf.
- Fifteen psychiatric hospital programs were equipped to serve deaf persons, but not one inpatient facility was available for the care of deaf children.
- There were 768 community mental health centers in operation, yet only one in the entire country was equipped to serve the deaf—in Fort Logan, Colorado.

In summary, it has been estimated that no more than between one and five percent of the mental health treatment needs of the deaf were being met.

The Story for Another Group

Hard figures on the mental health and treatment of persons with spinal cord injuries are simply not available. It is known that a large number of spinal cord injured persons live in social isolation. It has been estimated that somewhat more than a third of cord-injured persons suffer from serious forms of anxiety and depression. Morbid passivity is common. Drug and alcohol abuse levels are high. Between 12 and 50 percent of all deaths of spinal cord injured persons is by their own hand.

These estimates make clear that the spinal cord injured population has mental health problems. Furthermore, a study of whether psychiatric treatment would be helpful in the rehabilitation of seriously disabled children concluded that, "psychotherapy has a crucially important role to play in the total care of these [persons]." Nevertheless, the mental health professions give virtually no attention to the needs of this and other handicapped groups.

The evidence of this neglect is overwhelming: Beinecke's search of the literature in 57 medical journals over the last five years revealed no article published on the emotional health or treatment of the handicapped. What has been published can be found in nursing and rehabilitation journals.

No book addressed to mental health professionals on the subject has been published in five years. Of older books available on the psychology of the handicapped, not one is addressed to the handicapped themselves.

Other than various rudimentary and locally maintained lists, there is no national or state directory of services for the guidance of handicapped persons. In medical schools there does not appear to be any satisfactory training on the subject. No specific journal on the subject addresses either users or practitioners.

In short, there is not much information available on the mental health of the handicapped. What does exist is hard to find. When treatment is available, it, too, is hard to locate.

There seems to be a large amount of "denial" (in the psychological sense) going on—by society at large, by the handicapped, and by the mental health professions.

It is useful to ask why.

True, there is a category of psychologist specializing in rehabilitation. Although it might seem otherwise, these professionals are themselves part of the denial. They do little in the way of psychotherapy. According to Beinecke, compared to clinical psychologists, they spend four times as much time on such activities as "evaluation and assessment." Rehabilitation psychologists are placement officers, rather like counselors in high school. They are simply not equipped to treat mental illness. It may be that mental health therapists are reluctant to work with the chronically impaired. A study of those who work with epileptic people found that therapists experienced high levels of frustration and a sense of impotence. A survey of workers with the deaf found many felt "lost," inadequate to their task. Such feelings, it is interesting to note, are not unusual for professionals who treat *intractable illness*. This bespeaks a failure in the training of therapists rather than a necessary aspect of working with the seriously impaired.

A second reason for the failure to treat the handicapped is surely economic. The handicapped are often poor—poorer than other low-income people. They cannot pay much for therapy. Many are uninsured and not insurable—thus, mental health professionals cannot be certain of payment for their services. Eligibility for Medicaid does not help unless psychotherapy is provided in the coverage.

Lastly, as happens often in the case of the aged, treating disabled persons may not be seen as cost effective. The severely handicapped and the aged will not likely (it is thought) return to the marketplace. To expend the scarce time of a psychotherapist upon them cannot be justified.

Underlying these reasons, however, lies a base reason both somber and profound. Perhaps at the behest of society, the handicapped and the medical profession are engaged in a conspiracy. Rehabilitation, as currently practiced, is rather like a game of "let's pretend." The medical specialist works actively with the patient to replace—or to appear to replace—the missing parts. The concern is with the appearance of the thing.

By muscle training, by prosthesis, and by training in reading lips, the medical model "pretends" to make impairments disappear. The handicapped person strives to be "normal" and to see him or herself as "normal"; the doctor encourages this. Once propped upon braces or equipped with cane, and back at a workbench, the disabled person is "cured."

Normality has been regained. Implicitly, however, the medical model forces the handicapped person to repress or deny as "unhealthy" the genuine feelings of anger, hurt, and grief at any substantial physical loss. Thus, the very process of rehabilitation creates a built-in mental health problem.

In a similar sense, the popular movement for accessibility— although itself both important and healthy—can be seen as an extension of the conspiracy to encourage denial. The intent of accessibility awareness is to so adjust the environment as to make it possible for the handicapped person, using any combination of prostheses and other devices, to move about with approximately "normal" mobility.

Thus, too often I think, the effect of improved prosthetics, new technology, and advanced rehabilitation serves only to improve the quality of the pretense that the handicapped person is not disabled.

Psychiatry can have—and should have—no part of this pretense. In fact, what psychotherapy has to offer runs directly counter to this pretense. Psychiatry should seek to encourage handicapped persons to see themselves as they are in the world as it exists. It should encourage the acknowledgment of and coping with feelings—ugly as they may be—that are natural consequences of disability. The aim is to come to an accommodation with reality—and find an inner peace.

This is, after all, the work of psychiatry as commonly defined. The mental health profession should get on with its work.

From Manual
to Electric:
A Transition

Originally published in New Mobility, *March, 1992, this piece has been widely reprinted. Apparently it treats feelings that are widely shared within the disabled community.*

MY OLD MANUAL WHEELCHAIR is like the philosophy problem set by Grandpa's ax: "This is Grandpa's ax. Of course the handle has been replaced several times and this is the fourth new blade, but it is still Grandpa's old ax, isn't it?" My manual chair, an E & J Junior, is over 25 years old. Everything on it has been replaced two or three times—even the frame itself. The parts have been recycled but it is my same old chair, battered, hopelessly out of date, but *me.*

My old chair has taken me around the world. It once fell out of the trunk of a car going 70 miles an hour—and survived. In Africa it was stepped on by a hippopotamus. Jack Kennedy tripped over it in the U. S. Senate. In Alaska, my chair and I were lashed to a pallet and swung ten stories up and over the North Pacific onto an oil platform. I manipulate my old chair with a skill and precision borne of years of practice. My chair has been an integral part of my life, good days and bad, sickness and health, for more than a quarter century.

I am a polio: my trunk and legs are paralysed, my shoulders are weak, and my biceps and triceps are not so hot. Advancing age and "postpolio syndrome" are taking their toll. In recent years, I have lost muscle power and endurance. I must now carefully plan my outings, gauging how far my increasingly limited muscle power can take me. More and more, I have become dependent upon the push-power of my friends to get me out and about in the world. Incrementally, yet absolutely, I have become less independent, more invalid.

Clearly, time to think of an electric wheelchair.

I resisted the thought. Electric wheelchairs are for *crippled* people, not for folks like me. In my mind's eye, I am one of those lean, mean athletic wheelies who compete in the marathon and get their pictures on the back of Wheaties boxes. And besides, electric wheelchairs are *so big*, like Sherman tanks, nothing at all like my little lightweight chair, which goes so fast and turns on a dime. And besides, I want to be independent, I can't have my mobility threatened by battery failure. I am not the Energizer Bunny; I am flesh and blood.

Most reluctantly, I began the search for a suitable electric-powered chair. This took close to a year. There was something wrong with every model, every brand: too big, too high, too wide, too heavy, too expensive—all of them ugly to my eyes. Finally, thanks to the extraordinary helpfulness of the Invacare Company, I decided on an Invacare 9000, customized to the exact dimensions of my old E&J Junior.

I chose the 9000 because it has certain real advantages. The same size as my old chair, it does not impinge upon my independent lifestyle. I am able to make the same transfers and function in the same way from the new chair as from my old one. Also the 9000 is almost portable: the power unit pulls out and the chair folds. A reasonably strong and determined man can take it apart and put it in the trunk of a car in under three minutes.

It took time to get used to the electric controls. At first, I was a terrible, klutzy driver. I lurched around the house like a drunk in a dodgem car at the carnival. I took the bathroom door off its hinges, not just once but twice. I made holes in the walls. I upset a table and ran into a tree.

I had an attitude problem. Using the 9000, I had—still have—a sense of failure, a sense that I have given up, given in, after all these years of struggle, to my polio paralysis. I had a terrible feeling that, unless I continued to push my muscles each day to their very limits, they would soon waste away, leaving me not much more than a talking vegetable.

For the longest time, I kept the 9000 in the corner, using it only a few minutes a day. To my mind it was as seductive, dangerous, and habit-forming as drugs are for Nancy Reagan. The 9000 sang a powerful siren song: with it I could do wonderful things, things I have never been able to do in my manual chair. But I just said NO.

Here are some of the wonderful things I did with my 9,000.

I went to the National Gallery in my new electric. For the first time since polio, I was able to look at the pictures at my own speed without worrying about my own effort or fatigue or being dependent upon the sensitivity of the person pushing.

On my own, I went Christmas shopping at the mall, stopped for a drink and dinner, and then home again via a lift-equipped taxi van.

I went for hikes in my electric along the towpath of the C&O Canal National Park. This is a wonderful park that stretches more than 50 miles alongside the Potomac River. From the tow path I have seen turtles sunning, wild deer, a bald eagle and a rufous-sided towhee.

On summer evenings, often with my neighbor, I went for an electric stroll around our community, meeting and chatting with my neighbors for the first time.

I enjoyed all this greatly. It was a liberation for me to go out into the world independent of the strength of my arm muscles. I had not realized just how much in recent years my world had shrunk as my biceps had weakened.

Even though I have used a chair for 40 years, I am still self-conscious when I am out in public. I am still very aware how people react to me in my chair. It is my sense that strangers react slightly differently to me in my electric than they do to me in my manual. I think the manual is perceived as personal equipment—like crutches, or perhaps a blindman's cane. The electric, on the other hand is seen as a thing—a vehicle something like a golf cart. When you talk to someone in an automobile, he is *inside*, while you are outside. In a way, that is how people talk to me while I am in my electric chair: I am in my vehicle and they are outside it. My manual chair is not such an obstacle; it does not get in the way of conversation as my electric chair does. On the other hand, in motion, the electric chair moves from A to B so effectively, so efficiently, that it imparts to its occupant a dignity that is somehow missing in a hand-propelled chair. It is a *very sensible* way to go about your business.

I have had my Invacare 9000 for six months. It has changed my life. I use it full time around the house and I keep my manual folded in the back seat of my car. I no longer struggle with getting my manual in and out of the car. When I am going somewhere, I transfer from the electric to my car and leave the electric standing in the driveway. Using the electric I find I no longer have that deep, almost permanent muscle fatigue I used to drag around with me—or at least not so much. My arm muscles are more rested, and as a result I am able to do transfers better than I have in years. I also do more transfers. My arm muscles have gained strength yet may have lost something in endurance—but it is hard to say for sure.

In sum, I am not a failure, I have not given up, I am just sensible. I am *no* vegetable. I won't say I lived happily ever after, but I will say I have, at last, made the transition from manual to electric. It is a transition I should have made years ago.

SLAPPING UP SPASTICS

In the late 1980s, I began researching the German euthanasia program of the Third Reich. I was honored to be asked to present a paper on this subject at the First International Conference of Holocaust Scholars held in 1993 at the National Holocaust Memorial Museum, Washington, D.C.

I found that the museum, as originally designed, was not accessible to the disabled. When I arrived to give my paper on how the Nazi doctors had discriminated against and killed the disabled, I found that not only were there steps up to the stage, but also a flight of stairs into the auditorium. I raised a ruckus, the venue was changed and all went well. Since that time, the museum has undergone substantial retrofitting and, I am pleased to say, it is now thoroughly accessible to its disabled visitors.

I PRESENT THIS PAPER TODAY as the author of *By Trust Betrayed: Patients, Physicians and the License to Kill in the Third Reich*.[1] I am a historian; I

---

[1]*By Trust Betrayed: Patients, Physicians and the License to Kill in the Third Reich*, Vandamere Press, Arlington, VA, 1995. The book contains a full discussion, with references, of the issues raised in "Slapping up Spastics."

am also a severely disabled person, a polio quadriplegic. As such, I am interested in the evolution of social attitudes and assumptions toward disabled people. It is my conviction that the underlying assumptions that made possible the killing by physicians of upwards of 200,000 disabled German citizens in the 1930s and 1940s are still widely held, not just in Germany but throughout the western industrialized world. The purpose of this paper, as of my book, is to make the reader aware of these assumptions and of the evil that can arise from their careless application.

In the late 1930s and throughout World War II, physicians of Germany's medical establishment, acting both with and without the acquiescence of the Nazi government, systematically killed their severely disabled and chronically mentally ill patients. These people were said by their doctors to be "useless eaters," persons with "lives not worth living."

The officially sanctioned killing program was authorized by Hitler in 1939 at the request of leading figures of the German medical establishment. It was called the T-4 Euthanasie program, although most of its victims were not terminally ill nor in unbearable pain. They were not anxious to die. The program's proponents advanced various arguments for its justification—compassion, eugenics, economics, racial purity. The official program was halted by Hitler in the summer of 1941 in the face of a rising wave of protests from disabled people, their families and friends, and religious officials. Even so, many doctors, acting largely on their own counsel, continued killing patients in hospitals and institutions throughout Germany.

Over the course of the official program and the unofficial so-called "runaway" euthanasia which followed it, more than 200,000 German citizens met their death at the hands of their physicians. The mass murder techniques developed in the euthanasia hospitals were later used against Jews.

As part of the official program, the medical establishment was informed of the Aktion T-4 operation at secret briefings held across the country. At these meetings, the psychiatrists, physicians, and medical professors were fully informed on euthanasia. Euphemisms were used to describe the program: "negative population policies" were mass killings; "refractory therapy cases" were disabled people targeted for killing; "specialist children's wards" were children-killing centers; and "final medical assistance" was, of course, murder. There was never a doubt as to what was being discussed.

These men were told the euthanasia program was part of the "breakthrough campaign" necessary to obtain the new medicine of the Third Reich. This program held that medical attention and money should go, on a cost-benefit analysis, to those who can be brought back to full productive health. The chronically disabled would be removed from society as, said Dr. F. Klein, "I would remove the purulent appendix from a diseased body."

The "Reich Committee for the Scientific Registration of Serious Illnesses of Hereditary or Protonic Origin" was a high-level physicians' committee which met regularly with the Reich Chancellery. In the reports and minutes of the briefing meetings with rank-and-file-physicians, it was fiercely argued that the radical modernization of therapeutic activity could not be achieved without and, in fact, must go hand-in-hand with the elimination of these "refractory therapy cases." There can be no doubt that the existence and operation of the euthanasia program was general knowledge within the medical community of the wartime Reich. Throughout the life of the Euthanasie program—whether death came by pill, starvation, or carbon monoxide shower—it came at the hand of a physician. It was program administrator Brack's firm and oft-stated belief that, "the syringe belongs in the hand of a physician."

Bouhler, chief of Hitler's Chancellery, was insistent that a way of death be found that would be not only painless, but also imperceptible to the patient. He did not want to frighten the patients, nor make them uncomfortable. These things must be "done according to his orders, and in a dignified and not a brutal fashion."

The original regulations envisioned a "conservative" program with careful review procedures. In operation, the program became a matter of killing in wholesale lots. The psychological reasons physicians were willing to participate in these killings are no doubt complex. There is, however, an aspect of the structure of the program that made it easier. There was no single point of responsibility, no place in the procedure at which it was possible to say *here* is where the patient receives his death warrant; no point where it could be said, *this* physician is responsible for *this* patient's death.

The local practicing physician simply filled out questionnaires as he was required to do. The members of the assessing committee simply gave their individual opinion on each case. Nothing more would happen unless the members were in substantial agreement. The senior review physician simply went along with the committee or else expressed an objection. He was expressing a medical opinion, nothing more. Neither the assessors nor the review physicians ever saw the patient. The transportation staff was involved in transporting patients but it was no business of theirs where or why the patients were being moved. The staff that ran the centers were simply doing their jobs. Even the physician whose job it was to operate the gas chamber was not responsible for the death of the patients. After all he knew nothing. He had played no part in their selection; he knew nothing of their cases. He was only following the procedures laid down by superiors, carrying out the policy of the government as advised by the most eminent members of the medical profession.

The official, centralized euthanasia program lasted from 1939 through the summer of 1941. After two years of operation, the program's existence was widely known. The churches raised strong and vocal objections. There were public demonstrations in opposition to the killings. The German army was deep in the Russian campaign, and Hitler had no wish for public unrest at home. Accordingly, the Fuhrer, in a conversation with his personal physician, Dr. Karl Brandt, without ceremony or discussion, ordered a halt to the euthanasia program.

This did not, however, bring an end to the killing of the disabled and insane. Physicians across Germany continued to administer "final medical treatment" to patients they considered as having "lives not worth living." The killings continued, but the decision-making and the criteria used in these decisions became those of the immediate doctor, rather than the assessor committees and the review professors. The "children's campaign," by which retarded and deformed infants were put to death, proceeded unabated. Even *after* the war, U.S. Army occupation forces found the killing continuing at Kaufbeuren and Eglfing-Haar.

At the climax of the war, as allied bombing of German cities increased, Hitler made Dr. Karl Brandt health "czar" over all Germany. With his new authority, Dr. Brandt undertook to evacuate institutionalized patients to the countryside, where something on the order of 20,000 are believed to have been killed by their physicians. Physicians of another operation practiced wanton killing of the sick and disabled in concentration camps and occupied territories. On the eastern ramparts of Germany in Danzig, Pomerania, and West Prussia, as well as in Poland, mentally ill patients were simply shot by stormtroopers and the local police forces. What the Germans at the time referred to as "wild euthanasia" led to additional, widespread, disorganized, and indiscriminate killing. A German doctor, Hans Dorner, has said, "Unplanned groups and individuals were murdered: welfare wards, asocials, wayward children, healthy Jewish children, or those of mixed blood, homosexuals, political offenders, elderly wards of nursing homes, sick and healthy Eastern workers."

It is not possible to tell with any accuracy how many disabled German citizens were put to death during the Nazi years. No reliable figures exist for the spontaneous killings. Figures survive for the official centralized T-4 killings:

	1940	1941	Total
A (Grafeneck)	9,839	—	9,839
B (Brandenburg)	9,772	—	9,772
Be (Bernberg)	—	8,601	8,601
C (Linz)	9,670	8,599	18,269
D (Sonnestein)	5,943	7,777	13,720
E (Hadamar)	0	10,772	10,072
Totals	35,224	35,049	70,273

In the summer of 1991 unexpected verification of these figures was unearthed in the cellar of the headquarters of Stasi, the former East German secret police. The medical files of the 70,000 patients, filed alphabetically, were discovered by English scholar, Michael Burleigh.

In some of the Nuremberg trial documents, the figure 120,000 is given as the overall number of inmates killed in public institutions. According to German historians Aly and Roth, this number is on the low side and does not include those who died in such separate programs as the children's operation, random euthanasia, and the so-called "Brandt campaign." Dr. Leo Alexander, who served with the Office of the Chief of Counsel for War Crimes at Nuremberg who performed the major study of the euthanasia program for the court, has estimated that 275,000 persons were killed. The psychiatrist, Fredric Wertham, has looked into hospital records. He found, for example, that Brandenberg in 1938 had 16,295 mental patients from Berlin. By 1945, there remained but 2,379 patients. In an institution called Berlin-Buch, out of 2,500 patients, only 500 survived. Kaufbeuren in Bavaria had 2,000 patients at the beginning of the war, and 200 remaining at the war's end. Many mental institutions simply closed their doors because of lack of patients. In 1939, for all of Germany, there were some 300,000 mental patients. In 1946, there were 40,000. This is not to say that all these persons were destroyed by the German state in the course of its euthanasia operation. After all, the general German war losses were colossal. Nevertheless, it cannot be doubted that the euthanasia program swept out entire wards, cleaned out entire hospitals. It decimated the entire German population of the severely disabled and chronically insane. The Euthanasie killing program was no Nazi aberration. Rather it was the efficient application through public policy of the theories of leading Darwinian scientists and philosophers in Western society.

Darwin's theories of evolution combined with the rediscovery of Mendelian law had encouraged Victorians in the belief that the biological world could be as knowable, as predictable, as Newton's physical world. Social Darwinism and the "science" of eugenics sought to apply evolutionary and genetic principles, as understood, to human society and breeding. Eugenicists believed that most human characteristics were inherited. In W. Duncan McKim's book, *Heredity in Human Progress*, published in 1900, heredity is blamed for, among other things, ". . . insanity, idiocy, imbecility, eccentricity, hysteria, epilepsy, the alcohol habit, the morphine habit, neuralgias, 'nervousness,' Saint Vitus's dance, infantile convulsions, stammering, squint, gout, articular rheumatism, diabetes, tuberculosis, cancer, deafness, blindness, deaf-mutism, color blindness." It is, he said, "the fundamental cause of human wretchedness."

U. S. President Theodore Roosevelt spoke for many forward thinking people when he said, "Someday we will realize that the prime duty, the inescapable duty, of the *good* citizen of the right type is to leave his or her blood behind him in the world; and that *we have no business to permit the perpetuation of citizens of the wrong type*" (emphasis added).

The impact of Darwinian theory upon German thought was no less than in Britain and America. Darwin cast a long shadow over the development of national socialism and the Third Reich. Perhaps most influential was the 1920 book, *The Destruction of Life Devoid of Value*, written by psychiatrist Alfred Hoche and lawyer Karl Binding. These men were professors of reputation and importance. They argued that the medical profession should participate not only in health-giving, but also, in certain circumstances, in death-making. With a carefully reasoned argument, defining their terms precisely, their analysis concluded that certain people should be exterminated for racial "hygienic" purposes. They argued that the retarded, the deformed, the terminally ill, and those who were mentally sound but severely damaged by disease or accident should be put to death. They believed that the death should be painless and expertly administered, that is, by a physician. According to their reasoning, the right to "grant death" was a natural extension of the responsibilities of the attending physician.

Binding and Hoche were widely read and vigorously discussed. One of their readers was the young Adolf Hitler who had read a good deal on eugenics before writing *Mein Kampf*. On one occasion Hitler even allowed his name to be used in advertisements for Hoche's books.

There were numerous other books and articles on the subject. The romantic philosopher Ernst Haeckel's book, *The Riddle of the Universe*, sold well for many years. His disciple, Heinrich Ziegler was a popular writer on such issues and won the important Krupp literary award. The 1920 book, *Moral der Kraft*, by Ernst Mann advocated that disabled war veterans kill themselves to reduce welfare costs.

An exceedingly popular movie in the Germany of the mid-1930s dealt entirely with the issue of euthanasia for the disabled. *I Accuse* is the story of a young woman suffering from multiple sclerosis. Her husband, a doctor, after lengthy soul-searching, kills his wife in the last reel as a fellow physician in the next room plays softly and funereally on the piano.

Training films, long thought lost, illustrated the unbearable life of the insane with particularly grisly shots of defective dystonias. These films were made for the use of medical societies. They were widely shown to physicians' gatherings and shown to the Nazi Party Meeting of 1935 by Dr. Gerhardt Wagner, leader of the medical delegation.

Although long lost, the raw unedited footage of these training films and their original scripts were found in the basement of Stasi secret police headquarters in the summer of 1991 by Michael Burleigh. Making use of this material, Burleigh pieced together a documentary film, *Selling Murder: The Killing Films of the Third Reich*, broadcast in Britain in November 1991. It is a remarkable experience for the historian, who has researched the T-4 Euthanasie program for years, actually to see in operation the killing center at the Hadamar Psychiatric Hospital. While the researcher knows it *happened*, the films actually show it *happening*. The impact is extraordinary.

In the film script, a "professor" lectures that the "incurably mentally ill" have a "right to die." "Is it not the duty of those concerned," he asks the eager, note-taking students described in the script as "today's strong, racially pure and healthy youth." "Is it not the duty of those concerned to help the incapable—and that means total idiots and incurable mental patients—to their right?" This film is now available for researchers at the National Holocaust Memorial Museum.

The economics of euthanasia for the chronically disabled were widely discussed. It was wartime, budgets were sky-high, deficits were extraordinary, health resources were limited. It was argued that expenditures for long-term care of patients, who might never again be economically productive citizens, made little economic sense in cost/benefit terms as compared with similar expenditures on improved public health programs to keep the able-bodied healthy. Scarce health care resources were to be rationed.

This thinking was based on the assumption that the life of a disabled person was less valuable to himself and to the state than that of an able-bodied person. This general devaluation of disabled lives was wide-spread, even to schoolroom textbooks. One text, *Mathematics in the Service of National Political Education*, set the following problem: "If the building of a lunatic asylum costs six million marks and it costs fifteen thousand marks to build each dwelling on a housing estate, how many of the latter could be built for the price of one asylum?" Another asked, "How many marriage allowance loans could be given to young couples for the amount of money it costs the state to care for the crippled, criminal, and insane?"

When the German physicians and medical professors set up T-4 Euthanasie, they were instituting a program whose principles had been widely and thoroughly discussed.

After the war, Dr. Karl Brandt, director of the Euthanasie program and Viktor Brack, administrator of the program, were hanged at Nuremberg for war crimes and crimes committed against humanity. Many of the principal T-4 physicians fled or disappeared. Occasionally, one has surfaced and faced trial. These trials have been long and drawn out, unsatisfactory affairs, largely because of the unwillingness of one physician to testify against another.

Other principal physicians simply resumed their practices under assumed names. Their presence was known to their peers in the medical community, but was not reported. The rank and file of German physicians, those who had been active in the program and the rest who had raised no objection to it, continued the practice of medicine, albeit no longer killing their patients.

Over the half-century since the T-4 program, the German medical establishment has never offically acknowledged complicity in, or apologized for, the killings. There has been no compensation for the victims or their heirs. A book summarizing accurately the T-4 Euthanasie evidence accumulated in the Nuremberg trials, written by a young psychiatrist, Alexander Mitscherlich, was published in 1949. It was suppressed and denounced as ". . . irresponsible . . . lacking documentation." The book was seen an attack upon the ". . . inviolable honor of German medicine." One reviewer said that only a "pervert" would read such a book and called its author a "traitor to his country."

The German medical establishment retains, and rightly so, great prestige. German physicians have made many important contributions throughout the history of medical science. Unfortunately the German medical establishment has chosen to deal with the Euthanasie episode with what amounts to an across-the-board denial. Medical students have been expelled from medical schools for attempting to discuss the matter. It is reported that Dr. Harmut M. Hanauske-Able was no longer able to practice in Germany after publishing an article on the subject in the British medical journal *Lancet*, (1986). In 1977, the courageous Margarete and Alexander Mitscherlich wrote in the foreword to their book, *Die Unfahigkeit zu trauern* (*The Inability to Grieve*), "Today in many minds, there is a reluctance to accept the facts of history. . . . What happened in the Third Reich remains alive in our subconscious, dangerously so. It will be fatal for us to lose touch with the truth of what happened then. We must struggle to seek out the truth of that era rather than search for improved defenses to hide us from this truth."

Encouragingly in the 1980s, a new, younger generation of historians began to focus their attention on the social history of the Nazi years. In the course of their studies, they have done important research on the T-4 Euthanasie program and associated killing. This work is only now being published. These historians include Ernst Klee, Goetz Aly, Karl Heinz Roth, Benno Müller-Hill and Michael H. Kater. Their work documents the known killings and uncovers killings hitherto unknown.

A breakthrough of sorts occurred at the annual meeting of the principal German medical society, Deutsche Artzetag in 1989. In spite of heavy resistance, the Berlin Chamber of Physicians mounted an exhibit, "The Value of the Human Being," which portrayed the role of German doctors during the Nazi years. In conjunction with the display, articles on medicine in the Third Reich were published in the *Deutsch Artzeblatt*, the German equivalent of the *Journal of the American Medical Association*.

In his remarks opening the exhibit, University of Munster medical historian, Richard Toellner, said, "The . . . entire medical profession was involved and they all knew what they did. . . . A medical profession, which accepts mass murder of sick people as a normal-

ity, and to a large degree explicitly approves of it as a necessary, justified act for the sake of the community, has failed and betrayed its
mission. Such a medical profession *as a whole* has become morally
guilty, no matter how many members of the profession directly or
indirectly participated in the killing of sick people in *a legal sense.*"
(Emphasis added.) This set off a storm of protest. The chairman of
the national organization, Karsten Vilmar, asserted that the majority
of doctors had honorably served the medical needs of their patients;
they were not aware nor did they participate in the atrocities.

In Germany today, as in the United States, there is a lively, ongoing
debate over issues of health delivery and medical ethics. Present, like
Banquo's ghost, in all these discussions must be the memory, expressed
or unexpressed, of the medical killings of the 1930s and 1940s.

The rationale in the 1930s was grounded on eugenic "principles,"
Social Darwinism, and a humane concern for persons judged by
their doctors to have lives "not worth living." Then as now, budgets
were in deficit, health-care resources were limited, and rationing was
called for. Careful economic cost/benefit analysis led to the diversion
of funds from the treatment of "recalcitrant" long-term chronic
patients to patients more likely to respond positively to therapy,
more likely to return to full productivity. The health and well-being
of the *Volk* as a whole were of greater value than that of the individual unfortunate.

Today in Germany, as well as in the United States, similar economic concerns, similar budget constraints impact the health-care
debate. Valid questions are raised concerning such issues as the cost-
effectiveness and social merits of intensive life support care for the
terminal AIDS patient, liver transplants for the chronic alcoholic,
kidney dialysis for the aged, and lifetime care for the very high-level
neck and respiratory involved quadriplegic. Such matters as abortion,
amniocentesis, tracking the genome, "the right to die," euthanasia,
and disability rights are both complex and unavoidable. These are
brutal issues, inescapably requiring cost/benefit analysis and "quality of life" judgments, implicitly measuring the value of human life in
economic terms.

Sometimes these measurements become quite explicit. A troubling
example can be found in the debate over the cost of care for severely

disabled, premature neonates. *Der Spiegel* recently reported a doctoral dissertation that asserted that 7.3 million marks could be saved in the cost of care and special education for "each handicapped child not born." It concluded as much as 730 million marks could be saved if 100,000 "genetically damaged" babies were aborted. This study illustrates how easy it is for well-meaning, socially conscious debate to slip, almost imperceptibly, into the devaluation of the lives of the people being discussed.

Present today in this country and in Germany, just as in the Third Reich, are three underlying assumptions:

- Otherness: This is the assumption that we—our group however defined—is better than others. Christians are superior to Jews, whites to blacks, straights to gays, the able-bodied to the disabled, physicians to patients. The superior group, whether termed "superior" by reason of birth, wealth, education, or status, believes that its superiority gives it the authority to make judgments or take actions affecting the well being of lesser groups.
- Spread: This is the often unconscious assumption that a person, disabled in one way, is therefore disabled in all other ways. Because a child with cerebral palsy may be unstable on his feet, the assumption often made is that he will be unstable in his mental processes. If a disabled person cannot do one thing, it is assumed he cannot do anything—he is useless.
- Devaluation: This is the assumption, again often unconscious, that because a person is flawed, he is therefore without value. He is a devalued person, useless. Whether the person is aware of it or not, his is a life not worth living.

We know the unspeakable acts committed in the Third Reich because of these assumptions. I warn you to look about you at things happening today.

A particularly vivid example of this issue took place at Rehab 88, the fifth international rehabilitation trade fair, held at Karlsruhe in 1988. The keynote speaker for the professional section of the conference was Hans Henning Atrott, president of the German Society for Humane Dying. His subject was, "Active Assistance for Dying: The

Final Rehabilitation." It is perhaps not surprising that organizations of disabled persons were outraged that such a talk should be given on such an occasion. They protested to the conference organizers but to no avail. As a last resort, they broke up Atrott's lecture by bursting into the hall in their wheelchairs, dressed in garbage bags, sipping from cans labeled cyanide, and waving signs that read, "useless lives" and "lives not worth living." Atrott found it all most unfortunate, telling the media that the protest reminded him of Nazi tactics. It was a return, he said, to "terror against different thinking."

In unified Germany, the neo-Nazi bully boys have been abusing disabled people. The Nazi punks call it, "slapping up spastics."

People in wheelchairs have been spat upon, cursed, and physically attacked. The *Journal of the British Council of Organizations of Disabled People* reports that as many as 1,000 disabled German citizens have been harassed, physically or verbally, over the last year. The disabled have been taunted with shouts of "You are wasting my tax money;" "You are a worthless liver;" "Under Hitler you would have been gassed."

The national newspaper, *Der Zeit*, reports on a particular case, that of Mr. Guenter Schirmer. Mr. Schirmer, age 46, was paralysed by an auto accident 13 years ago. He lived in a small town near Hanover. He was able to move about on his own, making use of a tricycle-type of wheelchair. In a visit to Hanover, Schirmer was attacked by a large gang of neo-Nazis who spat upon him, kicked his wheelchair, all the while taunting him with shouts of, "Under Hitler, you would have been gassed!" The abuse had its climax when Schirmer and his wheelchair were thrown down a subway staircase.

After several episodes of such abuse, Schirmer, depressed, killed himself. In a suicide note to his wife, Schirmer wrote, "The handicapped are unlikely to have a chance ever again in this world. . . Under Hitler I would have been gassed. Perhaps all these young people are right." Devaluation is contagious.

These young people have been busy. The local Pestalozzi Foundation, which cares for mentally and physically disabled children, reports similar attacks on their clients. Elsewhere, five hearing-impaired boys in Halle were set upon by a gang of punks who beat them so severely they needed hospitalization. Group homes for disabled people have been attacked in Stendal and Quedlinburg.

It is not fair to lay all the blame for such events at the feet of the Nazi youth. On a Blind Awareness Day in Hanover, blind people were passing out pamphlets at a stall in the marketplace. They were abused and insulted by passersby. Parents of disabled children in Hanover protest that school authorities discriminate against their children, refusing to allow them on school trips. At Spiekeroog on the North Sea, handicapped children attending a church retreat were made to leave the beach by able-bodied bathers who objected to their disabilities. These same children were denied access to a museum and later were forced off a path because pedestrians refused to let them pass. The handicapped already receive too much help, complained one of the pedestrians.

Most well known was the recent case in which a court ordered a 10-percent refund to hotel guests who were made to eat in the same dining room with disabled people using wheelchairs. In making his decision, the judge said he agreed with the plaintiffs that it certainly must have been a "nauseating experience."

It is my impression the underlying psychological attitudes and assumptions concerning the worth and place of disabled people in society have not changed very much over 50 years. The social, cultural upheaval now underway both in this country and Europe and the brutal social decisions that cannot be avoided in the allocation of health care, make it vital—as vital can be—that the martyrdom of German disabled people at the hands of their physicians be examined, widely understood and not forgotten.

DISABLED AMERICANS: CIVIL RIGHTS ARE NOT ENOUGH

In the Reagan-Bush years, a conviction grew in the disability rights community that "welfare"equals enslavement. I am convinced that in the events leading up to passage of the American with Disabilities Act of 1990, there developed an unspoken agreement between disability leaders and the conservatives in Congress. The leaders said, "Give us our civil rights and we will not need 'welfare' anymore." And the conservatives replied, "Fine. Here are your rights. Now, don't come back for benefits." This kind of thinking has made severely disabled Americans extremely vulnerable to cuts in Medicare, Medicaid and so forth. I wrote this as an op-ed piece and it has been reprinted in several papers across the country. It was placed in the Congressional Record *by Congressman David Price (D, North Carolina).*

THE AMERICANS WITH DISABILITIES ACT is a new law guaranteeing the civil rights of disabled Americans. The civil rights laws of the 60s helped black Americans in their struggle to lift themselves from the oppression of segregation. In the same way, the new Americans with

Disabilities Act will help disabled people in their determination to obtain free and equal access to employment, transportation, education, and indeed, to all aspects of society.

Passage of the act is the culmination of the nationwide civil rights movement of the last two generations. By guaranteeing the rights of disabled citizens, Congress has acknowledged the right to be different. It is an acknowledgment that, as a people, we are, in fact, united by our differences. It is a call—and a pledge—to make the world safe for diversity. This is the symbolic importance of ADA. The hope and confidence from which it springs are very American; they are true to the ideals on which the American democracy is based.

The parallel with civil rights for African Americans is apt. Thanks in part to the effectiveness of laws against discrimination, increasing numbers of black citizens have joined the mainstream of American society. Civil rights laws, however, have been of little help to those African Americans who are trapped in the nation's urban ghettos. Young black men living in a drug culture, without family or education, without prospects or skills, need more than civil rights.

Conservatives in Washington have argued that passage of the American with Disabilities Act will allow disabled people to get off the welfare roles, take employment, and become tax-paying citizens. And so it will. Many of the disabled are already employed taxpayers, and many more soon will be.

However, large numbers of America's most severely disabled citizens will not. If these people take a paying job, they will lose the services—attendant care, health care, food stamps, and housing subsidies—which are theirs under present law as long as they have no income. There are not many entry jobs for severely disabled people that pay the $30,000+ required to make up for the benefits they would lose.

Also, under present law, if a handicapped person goes off the disability rolls to take a job, he is unable to regain coverage should the job not work out, unless he can prove a new disability. Few, indeed, are willing to take such a risk.

These are inequities, and they should be fixed. Even such reforms will not help the severely disabled people—good, decent, deserving American citizens—who simply are not able to work. The plight of these people is not relieved by pledges to end discrimination in the work place. The schizophrenic patient sleeping on the street needs more than civil rights; he needs a meal, a roof over his head, treatment, and concern. The old disabled lady with no funds, warehoused in a public institution, needs her rights, but she also needs the dignity that decent care provides. The severely mentally impaired and the multiple handicapped, and their family and friends who struggle to provide for them, need civil rights, yes; but they also need better support from our rich society.

ADA, like the civil rights acts of the sixties, will certainly encourage upwardly mobile, well-motivated, physically active disabled people to move into the mainstream. It would be perverse if, at the same time, ADA was used as an excuse by the nation as a whole to forget the needs of those who are severely disabled as it has forgotten the needs of the permanent underclass in the black ghettos of our cities.

"Benign neglect" has not worked for these Black Americans, and it will not work for severely disabled citizens.

GROWING OLD
WITH POLIO

The following piece was written at the request of my friend, Dr. Lauro Halstead. It is reprinted from his book, Post Polio Syndrome, *Lauro S. Halstead, M.D. and Gunnar Grimby, M.D., Ph.D., Editors (Hanley & Belfus, Philadelphia, PA, 1995).*

> "I'll wrack thee with old cramps,
> Fill all thy bones with aches, make thee roar
> That beasts shall tremble at thy din."

Prospero's curse of Caliban
SHAKESPEARE, *THE TEMPEST*

I AM A QUADRIPLEGIC POLIO[1] and a member of the first large-scale generation of seriously paralysed polios to survive into old age. Thanks to antibiotics, advancements in medical care, orthotics and good luck,

---

[1]The term polio is used throughout the text to denote a person who has a residual paralysis caused by the disease poliomyelitis. This is used in preference to such terms as polio victim, polio survivor, etc.

I'm still here. I have lived with my disability, independent and self-supporting, for more than forty years. And now, like many others, I find my polio-ravaged muscles are developing new weakness, new cramps, new aches; my energy and endurance are leaching away.

Whatever the cause of this—and there are conflicting theories—I must live with it. My problem, and the subject of this chapter, is how to maintain the quality of my life as I age.

How to deal with aging is a search older than Hippocrates. The problems faced by the aging polio are not different in kind from those of the aging able-bodied—but they *are* different, very different in degree. Age comes earlier, with greater impact to the polio. What is no more than annoying to the aging able-bodied can be totally disabling to the polio.

Everybody is different; everyone has different problems and they have different solutions. These problems have common threads and perhaps some of my own experiences will be helpful to other polios (and their health providers) as they work to resolve their own unique problems.

Here are five areas that I have found to be of particular importance to the aging polio—at least, to *this* aging polio: professional, economic, engineering, psychological and philosophical.

Professional. Doctors today know little about polio. With the exception of the older generation, now retiring from practice, and certain specialists in physical medicine, most of today's physicians have never seen an active case. The late effects of polio, their impact on the aging process, what is now generally called post-polio syndrome—these things are often unrecognised and misdiagnosed. Many polios have been ineffectively treated for conditions they did not have; just as many have been told erroneously that their complaints are psychological in origin and that they should seek relief in psychotherapy.

Today's polio, to the extent possible must act as his/her own chief doctor. Only I know what it takes for me to remain functional in my daily living. Only I know what impact bed rest has; what impact a hospital stay can have on my functional ability and personal esteem. Only I know, after many years of experience, the sort of reaction medications can have on my body. Only I know how to monitor myself closely. Only I have developed an early warning system to detect and deal with problems before they become major.

I do not mean that I know more of medicine than does my physician. Not at all. I know more about *me*. When I consult my doctors, they bring their knowledge of medicine to the conference, I bring my knowledge of my paralyzed body. Together we analyze what is wrong, what treatment is advisable and what its impact is likely to be—on the problem and on my ability to function independently.

I have found that once this approach is explained, physicians accept its premise and appreciate it. It is a burden to be the God-like, father-physician, making life or death decisions for the compliant, all-trusting patient. I have found that responsible physicians are willing, even relieved to share some of this burden. If your doctor does not accept this approach, find another doctor.

Economic. My muscle power and endurance are as coins in my purse. I only have so many and they will only buy so much. I must live within my means and to do this I have to economize: what do I want to buy and how can I buy it for the least possible cost? Shop around and plan ahead. In terms of muscle power and endurance, I can still pretty much go wherever I used to and do pretty much what I used to—but not as easily and not as often. I must assign priorities and ration my activities.

Growing old with polio is a matter of economics: cost/benefit analysis. How much expenditure of limited energy for how much satisfaction. Minimize the exertion; maximize the pleasure.

Polio-weakened muscles have a finite, lifetime limit. I know polios who refuse to accommodate their life style to their weakening muscle condition. They function on will power; forcing their muscles, without regard to pain or spasm, to do their daily duty as they have in times past. This is like spending down your IRA retirement account before you are dead. This can be a desperate game. One polio I know of, after years of "walking" on will power alone, killed himself rather than use a wheelchair. Others grumble but adjust as they move from braces to a wheelchair, from a manual chair to an electric.

In my own case, I no longer work 9 to 5 in an office environment. I work part time at home and live more modestly. I am poorer but life is richer.

Engineering. Most of us polios have struggled throughout our lives to be as independent and self-reliant as possible. Now after all these years, when we find we must accept more help, we feel a real sense of failure: we have fought the good fight—and lost.

In my own case, for many years I refused to admit that I needed an electric wheelchair. In spite of aches, increasing fatigue and an ever-narrowing range of mobility, I was determined to tough it out with my manual chair. Finally when I could tough it out no longer, when I was forced to transfer to an electric, I was surprised that the quality and independence of my life improved greatly.

Over the years there have been significant improvements in orthotics, equipment, electronics, public attitudes and accessibility legislation—all of it having the effect of improving the quality of life of disabled people. Lightweight braces; practical, even portable electric wheelchairs; dependable van lifts; personal computers; improved transportation practices for the travelling disabled; drive-in automatic teller machines; telephone grocery services; cable TV. These things and many more are ready at hand to make things easier for the ingenious quadriplegic. For the person with major paralysis it takes the inventiveness of a Rube Goldberg and the skill of an engineer if he/she is to maximize functional ability. There is usually a way—one way or another—to get something done.

The problem of severely limited muscle power and the resulting restrictions of mobility can be analyzed in terms of Newtonian physics: mass, inertia and the application of force. A knowledge of the uses of leverage, pivot points, inclined planes, centers of gravity—these are invaluable tools. I am fortunate to have had training in the principles of static and dynamic mechanics. These have stood me in good stead as I analyze how to get me—and my body—from A to B and back again. While this intellectual approach has been most helpful, I do not want to diminish the value of plain intuition. Most of us wheelchair users over the years develop a pretty accurate intuitive understanding of what will work and what will not.

The Rube Goldberg aspect is using what is at hand to do what must be done. I need to get something from the high shelf in the closet so I claw it down with a straigtened-out coat hanger. I carry an ordinary ice bag with me at all times—an unobtrusive, portable urinal. An old piece of cow hide, slick on one side, rough on the other, serves as a portable "slide board". A stick with an egg cup on its end allows me, after I have transferred into my car, to steer my electric wheelchair far enough away from the car to close the door.

There is a nice sense of satisfaction that comes from figuring out how to do something that did not seem possible. This is a satisfaction familiar to all polio survivors.

Psychology. My rehabilitation at Warm Springs was a remarkably positive experience. There was a contagious "can do" enthusiasm, not unlike the enthusiasm of a football team on a winning streak. We were *pumped.*

We encouraged ourselves in the denial of the extent of our impairment. Unwittingly, we taught ourselves to hide it and work like hell to overcome it. With polio, this approach was remarkably effective. Polio is not a progressive condition. Maximum paralysis occurs at the height of the critical stage of the disease; with informed exercise and care, over a period of months and years, the paralyzed muscles will regain—and *retain*—a significant degree of strength and function. At Warm Springs, we translated this into work hard, push the limit and you can make your muscles do what you tell them to.

For me, this approach worked well for many years. I used my will power to drive my severely limited muscle power. Now I find the game has an endpoint. No matter how much will power is applied, my muscles are worn out. They can no longer do what they used to—and when they do what they still can do, it is only with pain and vast fatigue.

And here I confront the central enigma of polio. If I give up and let other people do for me the things I usually do for myself, my muscles rest and I feel fine. But then, in a very short period of time, I lose what strength I have left and—soon enough—I can no longer do anything for myself at all. And then I don't feel fine at all. So there is no alternative: Use it or lose it. And so I soldier on, all aches like Caliban.

Warm Springs rehabilitation had another, rather more complicated aspect. This was a direct legacy of Warm Springs' founder, Franklin Delano Roosevelt. We were encouraged, we encouraged each other to maintain a heroic charade. We convinced ourselves that, as to our disability, we never thought about it, we were never bothered by it; we could, we would to do anything an able-bodied person did—or die in the attempt.

And die we almost did. As the body rebelled, the fake facade became harder, ultimately impossible to maintain. And yet we were loath to let it go. So much of our pride, persona, self-image was invested in this heroic charade. It was the way we saw ourselves. It was our shield. With it we were invulnerable; without it, what are we?

And the answer is, without it we are human. It is, after all, very tiring to be always indomitable in the face of all events, to persevere without complaint no matter what. This is far more exhausting than mere physical fatigue. Not only is this superhuman, it is pointless. Surely after all these years we have earned the right to be human, to complain, and if warranted, to so cry out with Caliban, "That beasts shall tremble at thy din."

It is a liberation at last to be honest with oneself and one's world. If the charade was a shield, it was also a wall. It kept us from being emotionally honest with other people—it isolated us from them. That is too bad because we have much to share with them.

A Philosophical Afterthought. Polios have a certain advantage over the able-bodied when it comes to aging. Polios know things the able-bodied do not. Polios have, perhaps, a certain wisdom.

Many of us have looked death in the eye. From our childhood, we have known what it is to lose control, to be helpless, to suffer pain, to be terrified. And yet—as William Faulkner put it, not merely to endure but to prevail.

And now Post Polio Syndrome provides a refresher course. This knowledge of ours—painfully learned—gives a unique perspective on aging. It brings us certain advantages and serious responsibilities.

The advantages are of two types. The restrictions imposed by age are not new to us. We already know to live with limited mobility, limited energy and chronic pain. We do not confuse the quality of our life with the quality of our tennis game. We know that happiness is not dependent upon activity nor is meaningful defined by trophies. A meaningful life may be hampered—but need not be defined—by pain or disability.

The second benefit comes from our familiarity with death. We know death; it is not the enemy it is to able-bodied people. Death is the end, but that is all it is. We know, better than most, that we need not panic over our own mortality. As we get older, as our polio-frail muscles give out, we are reminded again—and forcefully—how fragile a thing is well-being. Our understanding of the ever presence of death means that we do not defer living. If there is beauty and meaning, love and happiness, it is here, now, and nowhere else. More than most, we live in the now.

It is, as I see it, our responsibility to share this specialized knowledge of ours with able-bodied friends and family as they confront the reality that—as the Prayer Book has it—"In the midst of life we are in death."

Today, America's popular religion is something different: it worships youth and fitness. Proper diet and exercise seem to guarantee well-being. The miracles of modern medicine, glowingly reported in the media, seem to guarantee a long and youthful life.

When decrepitude, disease and death come—as inevitably they do—they come as a surprise. It is then that the able-bodied turn to us. It is then our responsibility to help them as they have helped us with our disability in the physical world.

Susan Sontag has written, "Everyone who is born holds dual citizenship in the kingdom of the well and the kingdom of the sick." As Virgil guided Dante through the Underworld so, too, can we polios guide our families and friends as they pass through the kingdom of the sick.

In the cacophony of the age in which we live, it is not easy nor is it common for a person to understand the pain and fear of others and to reach out to them. Yet now, it seems to me, we polios find ourselves in a position to do just this. This is our gift, if we will use it. By so doing we help others and we enrich and make more meaningful our own lives.

Confessions of a Former (I Hope) Super Crip

Coming to terms with my own reality allowed me to speak out more directly and more candidly. The following was published in New Mobility *in 1995.*

SO THERE I WAS in Darkest Africa. In fact, it was dark. The sun had just set and though the game park was closed for the night, I was wheeling down the path to the river where the hippos spent their days. All at once, the ground began to shake. I heard a *boom, boom, boom,* coming toward me from the river. Just in the nick of time, I wheeled my chair off the path into the tall grass. Thundering past me, so close their leathery skin grazed my wheelchair, came eight hippos in single file on their way to the pasture where they graze.

So there I was in Alaska, "The Last Frontier." Piloting my little plane, an Aerocoupe, I was flying over Cook Inlet. The great Alaska Range was to my back, the Chugach mountains straight ahead. I was returning to Merrill Field in Anchorage. And then my engine died.

244

Not only that, the electrical system failed as well and I found myself without radio contact. Very coldly, very calmly I assessed my situation. I did not have my wheelchair in the cockpit. The Inlet waters were icy. If I ditched in the water, I would surely die before being rescued. I remembered that the plane could glide approximately seven times its altitude. I estimated I could just about make the field—if I was lucky.

And I was, just. I did not fly the pattern, I came straight in without warning. I coasted to a stop just under the control tower. The controllers went crazy, waving their hands, trying to tell me to get my plane off the runway because there was a plane landing behind me. But of course I could not move.

So there I was in England for three years. Living in a room without central heating or running water, the washroom toilet a block and a half away, up a ramp and down a ramp. It was an old Victorian affair with narrow stalls and high square walnut seats on the toilet. It too was unheated. It was so cold that my legs turned blue in September, not warming until April. I did not take a bath or wash my hair for a year at a time.

So there I was, down by the trucks at the docks in Greenwich Village. It was three in the morning in the car, pulling my chair in after me, when the crazed junkie came at me. I got the door shut as he tried to break the window by pounding on the window with the butt of his hunting knife.

So there I was, the lion charged the car, roaring as it sprang at my open window. Desperately I wrestled with the handle trying to get the window up before I was roadkill.

So there I was in a dog sled, just north of the Arctic Circle. So there I was, carried in arms, past the honor guard, up the steps and into *Air Force One.* So there I was when the Soviet agent asked me to procure a top secret document, and there I was when the CIA asked me to go to the Congo. "The Soviets will never suspect that we have an agent in a wheelchair out in the black."

"There are steps at the door," exclaimed the Prince of Wales, "how on earth did you get in here?" "Oh, Your Royal Highness," I replied, "Through the garage and up through the kitchen." "You know, he mused, "not even Buckingham Palace is accessible!" "I guess that's why I've never been invited," I said, but not loudly.

So there I was, the only person in a wheelchair in all of Oxford, all of Claremont-Pomona, all of Capitol Hill, all of the White House. So there I was.

★ ★ ★

Doing these things—and many more—did not make me a Super Crip. It was how and why I did them.

They were wonderful things to do. Some of them were exciting, some were fun, all of them interesting. I would not have missed them for the world.

What I regret now is that I did them all out of desperation. Here I was, a nice young man who had a bright future, suddenly "struck down by the deadly disease," polio, back in 1952. What was I to do? First of all, I would not talk about it; I would not even allow myself to think about it. I would carry on just as if I had never had polio, just as though I was not using a wheelchair.

I did not want to know, did not even *like* disabled people. I hung out with the able-bodied. I was absolutely determined. By hook or by crook, I would compete with the able-bodied. Not only would I be as good as they, I would be better. I would work harder, go farther, achieve more, so help me God. And I guess I did.

It was at terrible cost to my person. I repressed or denied everything. I had no feelings; at night, I had no dreams. No sex. I simply ignored pain and fatigue. I did not allow myself to get sick. I took risks and did things no sane person would ever do. I lived in terror of collapse, of fear that the world would see how hollow I was. I had a million friends but I could confide in no one because, in truth, I had nothing to confide. When asked about my handicap (as it was called in those days) I would reply, "I never think about it, never think about it at all."

I continued in this desperate fashion, wracked with constipation and insomnia, until July 4, 1974. On that day, I bombed out of Super Cripdom. My body collapsed physically, and I plunged headlong into a deep and chronic clinical depression, which took me years to climb out of.

Since then I have learned a lot about myself and about the world. I have learned how very nice it feels to take care of my body and its needs. Nowadays I lie down when I am tired, and I baby myself when I am sick. I set my own priorities. I do what I want to do and not what the world thinks I should. In my old Super Crip days, I was afraid the able-bodied world would shun me if I let them see a weakness. I was very wrong.

So, if you are a disabled athlete, compete in sports and go for the gold. If you are a disabled politician, go for the White House. If you are a crippled car thief, steal cars. Do not be a Super Crip and waste time trying to compensate or obfuscate your disability. What the hell, it's part of you.

Since I bombed out of Super Cripdom, I have continued to have an exciting, reasonably productive life. The difference is that now I enjoy it.

THE LONELINESS OF THE
LONG DISTANCE RUNNER

I have used this as the basis of several talks to polio support groups. I do not believe it has been published before. Aging disabled people, like runners, struggle with every new and old disabling pain. The following piece discusses the parallels between the two groups.

NOT SO LONG AGO I was having dinner with fellow polios, Ann and Charlie McLauglin. With us was our able-bodied friend, John Townsend. As soon as we were at table, I began complaining to Ann and Charlie about my aches and pains and they began complaining about theirs. Noticing that John was left out of the conversation, Ann turned to him and said, "Oh John, you must be bored with all this complaining!"

"Oh," said John, "not to worry. I've known Hugh for ten years so I am used to it."

So let me begin with an observation. *There is nothing in the world polios love more than talking about polio with other polios.*

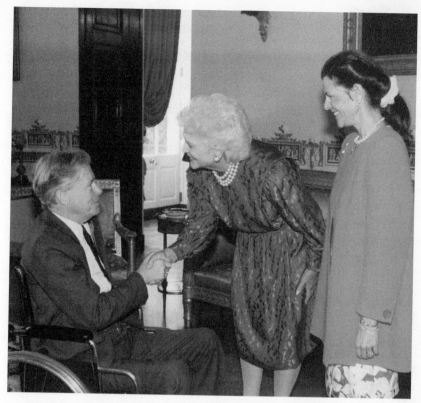

Tea at the White House with First Lady Barbara Bush and the Queen of Sweden in early 1989. The Queen had just published her book on sports and disability. I was a busy Super Crip.

A polio friend said the other day that when she first went to the polio clinic at the National Rehabilitation Hospital, she was told that, for a person with a pattern of paralysis like hers, the activities of daily living were as arduous as a marathon would be for an able-bodied person.

This set me thinking. We polio survivors are long-distance runners.

Long-distance runners are odd people. They are focused, even obsessed with their running. They run every day and neither snow, nor rain, nor dark of night will stop them.

They drive themselves to extraordinary feats of endurance. The ordinary marathon is the distance from the plains of Marathon to Athens, 26 miles, but today there are races with distances up to 100 miles.

Runners force their bodies to a level of strength and endurance far beyond their natural capacities. And as they age, it gets tougher and tougher for them to maintain this level but they keep at it. They never give up. They are stubborn people who refuse to accept their limitations.

And so are we.

Our muscles are paralyzed or partially paralyzed. Our muscular systems are able to function at only a percentage of normal strength. They have but a fraction of normal endurance. Nevertheless, we have taught them to perform marvelous feats. With exercise, ingenuity— and a good deal of chicanery—we have found ways to make our muscles perform what for the able-bodied are the ordinary, easy tasks of daily living. And, often enough, we have even found ways to make the way we do these tasks look normal, even easy.

In fact, they are anything but normal or easy for a polio survivor. And now, as we age, they get tougher and tougher. Like the long-distance runner, we are stubborn people who don't give up.

There is another, less obvious way we are like long-distance runners. It is our use of pain. The long-distance runner puts his body under great strain for long periods of time. If he is to achieve maximum performance and maximum efficient use of his energy, he must maintain all his body systems in top-notch condition. He must always *be aware* of what is happening in and to his body. To do this he must monitor body systems on a constant basis.

The runner is aware of his pulse, his heart beat rate, his blood pressure, his respiration, his fatigue. He knows the condition of his muscles, his joints, even his bones. The runner knows the usual aches, pains, and cramps that occur from the stress of the race. When these pains become out of the ordinary, when they become acute, the runner who wants to keep on running pays attention. Pain becomes his early warning system. The wise runner asks: What is this pain? Where is it located? What is causing it? Is the condition dangerous? Can I alleviate it or should I seek professional attention? And this is what we polio survivors do—or at least it is what we should do. We know all about the aches and pains. We drag them around with us on a daily basis. We don't like it but we live with it. However, when the pain is new, different, or persistently acute, we have come to learn that attention must be paid.

With the long-distance runner, failure to act on a pain signal could spell the end of his running career, but his daily life would not normally be threatened. With the polio, his career, his relationships, his very functional independence could be endangered by failure to monitor and assess changes in the pains and aches. In this sense, as they might say in Mr. Rogers neighborhood, "Pain can be your friend."

Why do people speak of the "loneliness" of the long-distance runner? Well, it is a lonely business. He must run alone for hours each day. He must run for miles and miles when his entire attention is devoted to nothing but assessing how efficiently his body is running. Even when not running, he is self-obsessed: diet, sleep, baths, and massages are carefully scheduled and analyzed.

Again, polios are like that. Perforce, we are self-absorbed, not to say self-centered. We have to pay attention to our body, micro manage our systems to a degree quite unknown to the able-bodied. Not many able-bodied people are aware of how much time and attention our bodies require if they are to remain in functional condition. This need to focus our attentions inward, to a degree of which the able-bodied world is oblivious, can make for loneliness. They may say they understand, but in many cases they do not. It is easy for a polio to feel all alone with his situation, to feel that no one understands. This too can easily lead to resentment and bitterness, which can cause an even greater sense of isolation.

This is why meetings such as this are so important—and so successful. We come together and compare notes. We learn what is new; how others deal with problems like our own; how to alleviate what can be alleviated and how to tolerate what cannot. We learn we are not alone. We get advice, empathy and support from each other. And so, let me close as I began: In all the world there is nothing a polio loves more than talking about polio with other polios.

CAN WE AFFORD
DISABLED PEOPLE?

I was invited to give the 14th annual James C. Hemphill Lecture at the Rehabilitation Institute of Chicago, September 7, 1995. The RIC is associated with the Northwestern University School of Medicine, and is arguably the best disability treatment center in the world. The invitation gave me an opportunity to address the perils of managed health care for disabled people. My lecture was published as a pamphlet by RIC and given wide distribution.

IT IS A GREAT HONOR to be asked by Dr. Betts to give the 14th annual James C. Hemphill Lecture. Mr. Hemphill was one of the founders of this unique Rehabilitation Institute of Chicago. This marvelous institute, built by the likes of Dr. Betts and Mr. Hemphill, is dedicated to the care and rehabilitation of folks like me. I had nine months of rehab at Warm Springs in the 1950s and it changed my life. I know from personal experience the work you do here is as important as any in medicine. It is based on love and respect and I salute you for it.

Not only is it a great honor, it is a rare opportunity for me to address a captive audience of health-care providers and I intend to make the most of it!

The title I have chosen for my lecture is, "Can we afford disabled people?" It is a dangerous question, dangerous because of its presumptions. It presumes that "we" are in a different category from "disabled people." Moreover, by asking it "we" presume to have the moral right and authority to answer it.

Speaking not as part of the "we" but as a person with severe disabilities, I think you will understand why I consider such a question dangerous. I reject it. I would argue the distinction between disabled and able-bodied is a false one. We are all a little bit able-bodied, a little bit disabled; and the degree we are one or the other shifts back and forth throughout life. As Susan Sontag has written, "Everyone who is born holds dual citizenship in the kingdom of the well and in the kingdom of the sick." I believe when one kingdom begins making life and death decisions concerning the other, society is asking for big trouble—and sure to get it. And yet in today's debate over the allocation of health dollars something close to this is happening.

Although I reject the question, I accept the issue: severely disabled people are expensive. They will become more expensive. With advances in medical high technology, the survival rate of severely disabled people will improve and the costs of their care will increase.

Other societies have addressed this issue and lessons can be gained from their experience. In the Germany of the Weimar Republic and the Third Reich, the question of allocating medical care to severe cases was asked and debated. Eminent scholars, writers, and physicians discussed the ethics as well as the cost of sustaining what they called life without quality, "life not worth living," i.e., the lives of severely disabled and chronically mentally ill people.

Before the Second War, the quality of German medicine was unsurpassed. Germany led the world in Nobel Prize winners for medicine and science. German citizens had benefitted from universal health-care coverage ever since Bismarck instituted a government reinsurance program in 1883. Health standards were very high.

It has been said that National Socialism—Nazism—was really no more than applied biology. So it is not surprising that with the rise of the Nazis came a new medicine ethic. Derived from social Darwinism and championed by public health specialists, the focus was on the health and well-being of the people as a whole. Curative medicine was to be replaced, announced health minister Gerhard Wagner, with preventive medicine.

The Hippocratic oath was old-fashioned. Physicians had a responsibility to their society as well as to their patients. Health-care dollars were scarce and a cost/benefit analysis must be applied to their allocation. Physicians providing treatment were expected to assess whether the costs of the treatment could be justified within the context of social policy. As a Dr. Helig said in a pamphlet, "It must be made clear to anyone suffering from an incurable disease that the useless dissipation of costly medications drawn from the public store cannot be justified."

In the late 1930s Germany's medical establishment asked for and was given the authority under careful and strict safeguards to provide what was euphemistically called "final medical therapy" for severely disabled and mentally ill patients who in the judgement of their physicians had lives "not worth living".

These safeguards did not last long.

The officially sanctioned part of the program, begun in 1939, was called T-4 Euthanasie, although most of its victims were neither terminally ill nor in unbearable pain. Nor were they anxious to die.

The official program was halted by Hitler in the summer of 1942 in the face of a rising wave of protests from disabled people, their families and friends, and religious officials. Even so, many doctors continued killing patients in hospitals and institutions throughout Germany.

Over the course of the official program and the unofficial so-called "runaway" euthanasia that followed it, more than 200,000 disabled German citizens, including many thousands of infants, met death at the hands of their physicians. Mass murder techniques developed in the euthanasia hospitals were later used in the Holocaust.

The Third Reich of the Nazi Germans was very, very different from today's America. Nevertheless it is my belief there was a "subtext" to the German killing program, a widely held—yet unconsciously held—set of social attitudes and priorities concerning disabled people that made the program possible. This subtext is not exclusive to Germany. I believe there is a subtext to the medical care debate in America today that bears a certain uncomfortable similarity with that of prewar Germany.

THE TYRANNY OF THE ABLE BODIED

In the Germany of the 1930s there was a nationwide fascination with youth and fitness and, as corollary, a devaluation of the old and disabled. The German people and their government were passionately dedicated to the proposition that it was the duty of each citizen to be healthy in mind and body.

To this end, there were campaigns against smoking, alcohol use, and unsafe sex. The importance of proper diet, exercise, regular checkups was emphasized. Vegetarianism, homeopathy, and holistic medicine were very popular.

For its part, medicine was to concentrate not on curing ailments but preventing them. Heavy emphasis was placed on keeping the healthy healthy. As Fritz Bartels of the Physician's League explained "The primary task of the physician is to discover for whom health care at government expense will be worth the cost." It was obviously a better use of these scarce health resources to restore a young, fit person to productive health than to treat a chronically disabled person with no hope of returning to a productive life. It was, of course, as the noted attorney Servatius later explained, a matter of humanity to fellow man: "Who would not have the desire to die while in good health rather than to be forced by all the resources of medical science to continue life degraded to an animal's existence! . . . Only misguided civilization keeps such beings alive . . ."

The United States today is at least as health-conscious as prewar Germany. Our nation is enamored with youth, fitness, beauty. It is the duty today of every right-thinking American to exercise, to brush, to floss, to eat low fat, low cal, high bulk, salt free, etc. If these things are done and done properly, one will never get fat or old, never get sick or die. And there is of course the corollary to this: If you *are* fat, sick, old or dead, it is your own fault. You did not take care of yourself.

Thus to a degree, if only subconsciously, the chronically sick or disabled person becomes the cause of his own distress. If the cancer patient had not smoked, if the quadriplegic had not taken the risk, if the AIDS patient had not done what he did, in short, it is his fault. Why should society be forced to support the endless and often astronomical costs of his care and treatment?

And in this way, the ineluctable hazards of illness and disability take on a moral quality.

DISTANCE DIFFUSES RESPONSIBILITY

Part of the effectiveness and success of the T-4 Euthanasie program was the manner in which therapeutic decision-making was removed from the primary care physician and passed on to—and diffused by—faceless committees, regulations and bureaucrats. Something like this is happening today in America as we move into health maintenance and managed care medicine.

This is how it worked in Germany. Responsibility for decision-making on whether to continue treatment of the disabled patient was removed from the attending physician. The patient's doctor simply filled out a questionnaire detailing the extent of disability, the length of treatment, the prognosis for recovery and return to useful employment, etc. The completed questionnaires went to a committee of respected physicians, each of whom separately reviewed them, deciding whether, in his judgement, the patient's prospects made him worthy of further treatment. These decisions were based upon guidelines prepared by public health doctors and administrators, based on economic and social as well as medical conditions. Only when a majority of the committee favored "final medical treatment" for a patient was his questionnaire forwarded to a review committee of senior medical professors. Only with their approval was the patient sent to a euthanasia center where a physician would administer death.

It is not irrelevant to point out that the review doctors and professors were compensated for their assessments. These payments acted as effective incentive to improve the efficiency of the assessors.

Committee doctors received 10 pfennigs per case reviewed, up to 500 cases per month. If the number of cases went over 500, the fee dropped to five pfennigs per case up to 3,000 cases per month. Take Hermann Pfannmuller as an example. He was a practicing pediatrician and director of a large Munich hospital. Even so, he found time to process in 15 months 159 shipments of between 200 and 300 questionnaires each. So efficient was Dr. Pfannmuller that he passed final medical judgement on 2,058 patients over an 18-day period!

The Germans knew what the managed care companies are learning, the money incentives work as well in medicine as they do anywhere else.

The key to the success of this hierarchical system of decision-making was the diffusing and distancing of responsibility. No one physician could say, "I caused this man's death." No doctor was forced to look into his patient's eyes and say, "Now I will kill you." All along the line, responsibility was ducked: "I simply filled out a form;" "I only gave an opinion," "I only helped draft the guidelines;" "I just carried out the order;" "The decision was made by physicians far more senior than I."

Something very close to this is happening in American medicine today. With the rise of health maintenance organizations, nationwide for-profit health-care corporations, and the increased power of the insurance companies, capitalism and cutthroat competition have come to medicine in a big way.

The competition is for the healthy person, the fit person, the one with predictable low medical maintenance costs. The practice is called "skimming." These standard, conforming patients with their predictable standard illnesses receive standard treatments and go about their business. The seriously disabled, the chronically ill person, especially the person with multiple maladies, the one who does not conform to the healthy profile is increasingly denied the extended treatment he or she needs.

I cannot give you statistics because they do not exist. There is no national index of the quality of care. I can, however, give you some examples that have come to my attention lately. I am sure you can add examples of your own.

- In an eastern city, newly spinal cord-injured paraplegics are denied treatment in an acute care rehabilitation hospital. You must be quadriplegic for that.

- An elderly woman in Connecticut who has been treated for stroke is sent home with stage IV decubiti, a systemic staph infection and impacted bowel.
- A young man with a stroke in Colorado is estimated to have an 80% chance of recovering his speech with four months of therapy; his insurance allows but four days.
- Stanford denies a heart lung transplant to a woman with Down's syndrome. The denial is without examination, made solely on the basis of her disability. The woman is a high-school graduate, who holds a job, lives alone, and is a respected leader in the disability rights movement.
- In New England, an obese woman is denied hip replacement surgery on the ground she will just wear out her new joint.

These patients are victims of managed care. Managed care is rationed care. Treatment decisions are no longer made solely by the primary care physician. Pretreatment approval must be attained from the health-care companies. Approval or denial is given by low-level clerks without medical training, making use of guidelines provided to them. These are regulations based upon standard costs for standard treatments. Unique conditions, particular to the individual patient, are not allowed for.

These regulations are drawn up by committees of physicians and statisticians, who are paid by the companies. The companies are profit-making and every effort is made to maximize their profit. Employees are offered incentives and promotions to increase cost-saving and profit-making. The motivation driving the employees is the profit of the company not the well-being of the patient. In fact no clerks, committees, or indeed, executives ever see the patient. They never look into his eyes and say, "I deny you the treatment you need." As in Germany, responsibility is distanced and diffused.

Under managed health-care, the primary care physician is the gatekeeper. The patient pays the HMO for his doctor's professional services, yet he is paid by the managed care company. The doctor has a fiduciary, to say nothing of a professional, obligation to provide his or her patient the best care possible. Yet, he is an employee of a profit-making company. He must serve two bosses. There have been cases in which the doctor is not allowed to inform his patient of therapy alternatives because of their high cost. There have been cases where the gatekeeper has not been allowed to refer his patient to a specialist even though a referral is clearly indicated. Such restrictions violate the physician's fiduciary responsibility to the patient as well as professional obligations.

I read recently of one HMO with surgeons on its staff. The company has calculated that for a particular procedure the standard hospital stay is X days. If the surgeon is able to discharge his patient a day early, then the surgeon gets the savings added to his salary. If, however, complications keep the patient in hospital longer than the standard stay, the surgeon's salary is docked accordingly. How anxious would one of these surgeons be to operate on someone like me?

The doctor of old treated his patient and the patient's family throughout their lives. The doctor was a part of the community; a part of the extended family. He made house calls, he had time to listen. He knew his patient. He had no miracle cures but he treated the whole patient.

Before modern times, the role of the physician was largely limited to seeing that the patient was comfortable as the body proceeded to heal itself, or not. In a very real sense, it is only in the last several generations that the physician has had the tools to "save" lives.

Medicine has changed completely in our lifetime. Today's America is a land of ever-increasing mobility. The family is fracturing and people are rootless. Today's physicians are busy, immersed in red tape and regulations. They specialize and they do not know their patients. They know their specialties. The advent of HMOs and managed care separate yet further the physician from his patient. The specialist sees the disease, not the patient. The HMO sees the expense and, often enough, no one has the interest, time, or money it takes to tend to the emotional and medical needs of the patient as a whole.

This is a situation fraught with danger for the person with a severe disability for, as we know, adjustment to a severe handicap has emotional and social components fully as important as the physical. Adjustment takes time and attention to the whole person. To ignore this may save money in the short run but only in the short run.

Unfortunately, the short run is the time frame in which the managed health-care companies operate. After all, it is the bottom line, the annual profit-and-loss statement that impacts stock value and management remuneration plans. The managed care companies are not interested in long-term care cases and are trying to, and succeeding at, pushing as many as they can over onto Medicaid and Medicare, thus raising the costs of those programs ever higher.

WHOSE DECISION IS IT, ANYHOW?

The physicians of Germany and the bureaucrats and their regulations were willing to make "quality of life" decisions. They presumed that their superior training and the prestige with which they were held by society qualified them to determine whether the worth of a patient's life was equal to the effort necessary to maintain it. Back in the 18th century, German physician Christoph Hufeland warned, "If the physician presumes to take into consideration in his work whether a life has value or not, the consequences are boundless and the physician becomes the most dangerous man in the state." What happened to the disabled citizens of Germany in the 1930s and 1940s illustrates, in stark intensity, just how dangerous.

However, treatment decisions must be made, and are made, all the time. It is instructive to see how differently these decisions are perceived by those who make them and those who are affected by them. In a recent study, emergency room physicians were asked: Would they wish to be resuscitated if this meant they would be left as high-level quads. Over 70 percent said no. When the doctors were asked to evaluate the quality of their present lives, 80 percent said pretty good. When they were asked to evaluate what the quality of their lives would be with quadriplegia, 82 percent said the quality would be pretty low. Then, a group of persons with high-level (C4 and above) quadriplegia for five years or more were asked to evaluate the quality of their lives and the same percentage as the doctors answered pretty good. When asked whether they regretted being resuscitated a smashing 92 percent answered no.

The physician, who fights illness and fears disability, and able bodied persons are apt to have a very different appraisal of the quality of life of a disabled person or an AIDS patient than does that person himself.

The behavior of the German physicians took place in Nazi Germany where, as has been said, "killing was in the air." Physicians, however, are only human and the assumptions concerning the quality of life of disabled persons made by the Germans can be found just beneath the surface, wherever you look.

Take, for example, a 1990 "Study of the Readiness of Jewish/Israeli Students in the Health Professions to Authorize and Execute Involuntary Mass Euthanasia of 'Severely Handicapped' Patients." Ninety-two medical students were asked to consider a hypothetical situation: You are on the staff of a well known Israeli treatment center directed by professionals of the highest calibre. Your patients are physically disabled, mentally ill or mentally retarded Israelis. Because of "a severe economic depression" followed by war, resources are becoming ever more scarce.

In a series of questions, the students were asked if they would participate in, at first, reduction of treatment of the disabled so as to "conserve maximum resources for the general population." They were then asked to classify the disabled to determine those who would benefit from treatment and those who would not. As resources become extremely limited, they were asked to "drastically curtail" treatment of the unresponsive disabled patients, and then, to participate in planning "euthanasia (mercy treatment)" for the "severely disabled so as . . . to end their suffering." Finally, they were asked "in order to carry out the euthanasia program in the best and most humane ways" actually to participate in the killing. The study found that 38 percent of the medical students agreed to curtail treatment of disabled people; 12 percent agreed to plan euthanasia for them; 9 percent agreed to carry it out.

At the Nuremberg Trials, Dr. Servatius defended the system under which physicians killed their patients. We remember him asking, "Who would wish to continue life degraded to an animal's existence?" A not altogether different sentiment is found in the American Thoracic Society's code of ethics. It says that life support ". . . can be limited without the consent of patient or surrogate when the intervention is judged futile." This statement is based on the physician's judgment that intervention would be futile. The Society helpfully defines futile as treatment: ". . . that would be highly unlikely to result in a meaningful survival of the patient." Again, that is meaningful as defined by the physician. As we have seen, the physician, to say nothing of the for-profit hospital or the managed health-care company, may have a very different definition of what is meaningful and what is not.

Meaningful life is an ineffable thing. It is not determined by how young, how rich, how fit, how beautiful you are. It is not even determined by how sick or disabled you are. We all know that some of the most valuable, meaningful of life's experiences can come in the midst of—even because of—pain and terminal illness. Quality of life is not something that someone else should be weighing for you.

However, treatment decisions must be made. Serious disability is an expensive business. The United States is by far the wealthiest nation on earth, the wealthiest in history. Nevertheless, as this wealth is now distributed, it is undeniably true that health dollars are limited and decisions must be made. As a nation, we have just begun a major struggle to determine how much, where and to whom Federal health funds shall be allocated. As Al Jolson said so memorably, "You ain't seen nothing yet!"

The outcome of this struggle will determine what kind of nation we are and what sort of society we wish to become. The signs are disquieting. As in the Germany of the Third Reich, voices are being raised questioning the expenditure of scarce funds to, as the Dutch Royal Medical Society has called it, "keep people alive too long." These are the people described by ethicist Peter Callaghan of the Hastings Center, as "biologically tenacious."

With the best intentions in the world, some of the participants in this national debate have been too willing to divide people into categories, too quick to set rules for these categories. Individuals do not fit into categories and their lives cannot be governed by some sort of abstract formulation of ethical standards.

Here are recent examples of how easy it is to get it wrong. Ethicist Earl Shelp sees severely disabled people as "dependent beings." He warns us of the ". . . tyranny of the dependent in which the production of able persons is consumed by the almost limitless needs of dependent beings."

Jeffrey Lyon, who is in sympathy with Shelp, admits that there are people with severe disabilities who do lead happy and productive lives but, he points out, these are the exceptions—these are what he calls the "dynamic, overachieving supercripples." Social policy must not be based, he insists, upon such exceptions.

The Hastings Center, among others, has tried to establish "Guidelines on the Termination of Life Sustaining Treatment and the Care of the Dying." There is indeed a problem here that deserves study. However, we are confronted by an enigma: As soon as we begin to think the unthinkable, the easier it becomes to think it. For example, among the categories of patients judged eligible for termination is "the patient who has a . . . disabling condition that is severe and irreversible." This thought has been taken a step further in the Netherlands where paraplegia and quadriplegia are now accepted as reasonable causes for physician-assisted suicide. Callaghan recognizes that such thinking might be difficult for some people: "There has been," he says, "a justifiable reluctance to exclude 'borderline' cases from the human community." This reluctance, he says could be overcome if, in our discussion of the subject, we are careful to avoid the excesses of the German physicians of the Third Reich who "spoke all too readily of 'a life not worth living.' "

Richard Neuhaus, Director of the Rockford Institute Center on Religion and Society, was perhaps not all wrong when he observed, in America today, "Thousands of medical ethicists and bioethicists, as they are called, professionally guide the unthinkable on its passage through the debatable on its way to becoming the justifiable until it is finally established as the unexceptionable."

Certainly medicine is changing. Traditional systems of treatment, service and payment cannot survive much longer. There are so many new therapies, so much new technology, the ability of medicine to understand the body and to manipulate its operation is advancing so quickly, that it outpaces the ability of present systems to cope. The demand for medical services of all sorts grows almost exponentially. So do costs. Demand and the costs thereof are rising so fast that there must needs be revolutionary change in the allocation and distribution of health care.

How these changes are to be made, what form they are to take is beyond my ability to predict. The process will be rough; it always is.

There will be injustices; there always are. But medicine is a noble calling and I am sure that, one way or another, it will continue to serve and protect its patients.

The point I wish to make today, to make as clearly and forcefully as I can, is that as these changes come about, those who make them, whether in the profession, private enterprise or public service, should keep always in mind these lessons of the German experience:

- There exists a false yet subconscious devaluation of people with disabilities and chronic illness. In fact, the lives of disabled people are no less valuable and need be no less satisfying than the lives of the able-bodied. Physicians and policy makers must never forget this.
- "Experts" who are qualified to make decisions in their field of expertise too easily come to believe their specialized knowledge gives them the authority to make "quality-of-life" decisions concerning the less powerful. These are in fact moral judgments rightly made by the individual involved.
- The removal of therapeutic decision-making from primary care-givers to economically driven management should be resisted. The farther away from the patient these decisions are made, the more dangerous it is for the patient. It is easier to authorize "final medical therapy" for someone you don't know, particularly if the responsibility for the decision is diffused throughout a bureaucratic maze of regulation and committee.

The point I make today is best stated by a member of another profession. During the 1930s criminal trial of Murder, Inc., the prosecutor asked one of the professional killers how it felt to murder someone. In answer, the killer asked the prosecutor how it felt to prosecute someone. The prosecutor said at first he was nervous, but he got used to it. "It's the same with murder," said the killer. "You get used to it."

LIFE IS A BANQUET

This is the text of a talk I gave to students at Ramapo State College, a part of the New Jersey University system, in the fall of 1995. It was one in a lecture series on "My Life is My Message."

CAESAR WROTE, most famously, "All Gaul is divided into three parts." So, too, my life.

For the first 20, I was able-bodied. I was ambitious, enthusiastic, and confident. In 1952, I had polio and became quadriplegic.

For 20 years thereafter, I lived a life of action and achievement. I tried to be the same person I was before polio—just as confident, enthusiastic, and ambitious. At the same time, I denied both the extent of my disability and the intensity of my feelings about it. As a result of this conflict I began my descent into an extended and severe situational depression in 1972.

For these last 20 years, I have lived a different sort of life and, I think, a better one.

These two great events—polio and depression—have shaped and tempered me, as steel is hardened in a fiery furnace. I am scarred as concentration camp survivors are scarred. But like them, I have learned some things about life from my experience.

I will tell you some of these things, but I do not expect you will hear them. You will hear me, but you will not understand what I am saying until you experience them. As I suppose, each in his own way, over the course of a lifetime, will indeed experience them.

There is a line in a Bob Seager song I often think of: "I wish I didn't know now what I didn't know then." Life would be so much easier that way, all sunshine and buttercups. But life is a learning process, and with this knowledge, painfully obtained, there comes a kind of wisdom and understanding that is precious.

DEATH—HAVE NO FEAR OF DEATH.

At the very climax of my struggle with polio, I had what is now called "an out-of-body experience." This was more than forty years ago. I had never heard of such a thing: certainly there were no books or articles on the subject. I had no name for what I experienced. I told no one at the time about it, and it was only many years later that I discovered that others, too, had experienced it.

I was dying. I had asked for and received last rites. I had said good-bye to my parents. My temperature was very high; my body was shutting down, the paralysis was advancing upon my brain. And then, I found myself—the essence of me—"floating" above my corporeal body. I could observe what was happening to me; I could observe my reactions, my conversation with others, my very thoughts—but I was not there, somehow. Or I was both there and above there.

There was a cave, a warm, protective cave, with a warm glow just beyond the mouth of the cave. For hours (days?), I hovered just inside the entrance, warmed by the cave. In the cave, there was no pain, no sickness—just warmth and protection. When called upon, I would come out of the cave to respond to a nurse or a doctor, but then I would return. I knew with a great certainty that I would be safe in the cave and that I could stay there forever if I just went deeper into it.

As you can see, I did not go deeper into the cave, and I am with you today. But ever since that day, I have known that death is nothing to fear. There may be much to fear in life, but there is nothing to fear in death. Death is a release and a reward.

DEATH—A FALL-BACK POSITION

When I was in the iron lung, breathing pure oxygen through a tube in my throat, paralyzed from head to foot, unable to swallow, with virtually all bodily functions shut down, I learned that dying was easy and that I could die at will. This was, and remains, a great, sustaining comfort to me.

If the pain—and there was a great deal of pain—should become too great, I could just let go and die. If my situation should become too hopeless, if my dependency on others should become too much to bear, I could just let go and die. For two months at least, this was literally true. Continued living was an act of will. Gradually, as my strength returned, this was no longer true. But the principle remained: I may be paralyzed; but if the party gets dull, I have the choice to leave at any time. I retain control. Remember that old Victorian poem, "I am the master of my fate. I am the captain of my soul." Well, it's true.

PAIN—YOU CAN TAKE IT

I had a great deal of pain, and I was given nothing to alleviate it. The pain killers available in those days acted to deaden the central nervous system and the breathing response. Even with an iron lung, tracheotomy, and pure oxygen, I needed whatever bit of breathing response I had left. To keep alive, I had to bear the pain. I did so, even undergoing surgery without anesthesia.

I learned about pain in those early days. There is no physical pain that is not bearable. Under massive and extended pain, a person somehow learns to tolerate, no, to endure it. You somehow retreat into yourself and dull down. The emotions and feelings, to the extent possible, are battened down. Like a voyage on the North Atlantic, the sky is grey, the sea is grey, life is grey and endless. It is cold comfort, but comfort nevertheless, that should the pain become too intense, you pass out. Of course, when you come to, the pain is still there, but you have escaped it, if even for a short time.

So, remember: pain is awful. It makes you miserable, but do not be afraid of it. Do not avoid doing what you want to do because it might be painful.

Breakdown

Before my depression, I had lived my life according to the expectations of others—peers, parents, teachers, doctors, bosses. I more than met those expectations. I had some crazy idea that if I did everything everybody wanted, then they would leave me alone, and I could at last be myself—do what I wanted, which was to write. That approach did not work. My physical and mental collapse in the 1970s was proof of that.

I had been using all my strength to maintain a facade of success and happiness. I had no life of my own. It had become harder and harder to repress my feelings of rage, self-pity, and despair. My life was killing me. I had to change it, or I would die. I did change it, but at great cost.

On July 4, 1974, I went home from my office and never went back. I crashed. For the next several years, I endured bleak depression, anxiety storms, panic attacks, amnesia, seizures. You name it; I had it.

Several times, I was very close to suicide, but curiosity saved me. As an old Jewish proverb says, "A man should go on living, if only to satisfy his curiosity." This is what I did. The Nixon Watergate scandal was reaching its crisis. Day after day, *The Washington Post* would have the latest revelation from its informant "Deep Throat." The hearings were producing unbelievable revelations about the President and the sleazy activities of his White House "Plumbers." I despised Nixon; I love gossip, and I am a consummate political junkie. Late at night, whenever I was about to kill myself, I would think: "Hey, wait a minute. What will be in the morning *Post*? Have they found the smoking gun? Are they going to impeach Nixon?" So, I would put it off; I just had to see what would happen next.

BREAKTHROUGH

R. E. Laing, the controversial psychiatrist, once wrote, "Madness need not be all breakdown. It may also be breakthrough. It is potential liberation and renewal as well as enslavement and existential death." This is, I think, what happened to me.

Gradually—over years, not months—with the help of analysis, religion, and, for me, the great art that is available in Washington, I became my own self, a person in his own right, and that person is a writer.

This process of self-discovery cannot be taught. It is very simple, yet very hard. You can encourage others to it, but you cannot lead them. Much of our society conspires against it.

Yet, it is the message of the ages. You read it in the Bible; you see it on T-shirts. Ricky Nelson says, "You can't please everyone; you've got to please yourself." Shakespeare's Polonius says, "To thine own self be true." Socrates said, "Know thyself." God, himself, in the first great commandment says, "Love thy neighbor as thyself."

LIFE—LIVE IT

When the English novelist Sybil Bedford turned 60, she had a revelation. She said that she had led her life so far as though in some manner it was a rehearsal, as though the play itself had not yet really begun. She was shocked at 60 to discover that it was *not* a rehearsal; it was the play itself. Not only that, the play was well into its third act.

Or to put it more succinctly, as an old psychiatrist said to a friend of mine, "Life is once around the block, Johnnie."

"Life is a banquet," said Auntie Mame, "and most poor suckers are starving."

I tell you, go to the banquet.

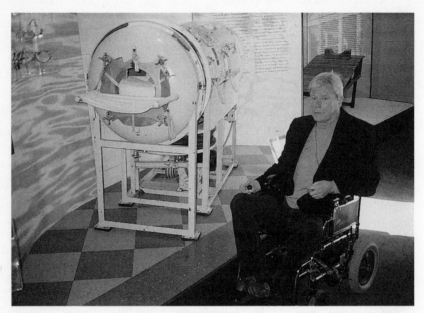

Forty-six years ago, I lived in an iron lung identical to this one. It was a shock to find it on exhibit at Warm Springs in February, 1998.

Photo by Dee Mullen

AFTERWORD

FORTY FIVE YEARS AGO TODAY I entered Bryn Mawr Hospital. I did not expect to stay long for I had a term paper due on Monday.

The subject of the paper was "Kant's Categorical Imperative." I never finished it. Now, perhaps, it is time to do so.

My life has been full. Happiness is made, said Freud, of love and work. I have had my share of both. I have tried always to learn all I could, to be as fair as possible, and to treat all men with honor and honesty.

There is but one categorical imperative says Kant. It is that your moral princples be only those you would wish to see become universal law. If there is one principle that has guided my life, one lesson that I would wish to become universal, it is this:

Alfred Tennyson's poem, "Ulysses," tells of Homer's hero, Odysseus, home from the sea. Blown off course on his way back from Troy, he has wandered the world and its wonders for some 20 years. An old man, back in Ithaca at last, he finds it hard to settle down. He wants to sail again, west to unknown lands. He may be old, he says but, "Some work of noble note, may yet be done."

Gathering his old crew together, he entreats them:

> "Tho' much is taken, much abides; and tho'
> We are not now that strength, which in old days
> Moved earth and heaven, that which we are, we are;
> One equal temper of heroic hearts,
> Made weak by time and fate, but strong in will
> To strive, to seek, to find and not to yield."

So like Odysseus I will continue. "To strive, to seek, to find and not to yield."

May 10, 1997
Cabin John, MD

INDEX